Countertransference Issues in Psychiatric Treatment

Review of Psychiatry Series
John M. Oldham, M.D., and
Michelle B. Riba, M.D.
Series Editors

Countertransference Issues in Psychiatric Treatment

EDITED BY

Glen O. Gabbard, M.D.

REVIEW OF PSYCHIATRY VOLUME 18

No. 1

American Psychiatric Press, Inc.

Washington, DC
London, England

Note: The authors have worked to ensure that all information in this book concerning drug dosages, schedules, and routes of administration is accurate as of the time of publication and consistent with standards set by the U.S. Food and Drug Administration and the general medical community. As medical research and practice advance, however, therapeutic standards may change. For this reason and because human and mechanical errors sometimes occur, we recommend that readers follow the advice of a physician who is directly involved in their care or the care of a member of their family.

04 03 02 01 5 4 3 2

Manufactured in the United States of America on acid-free paper

American Psychiatric Press, Inc.
1400 K Street, N.W.
Washington, DC 20005
www.appi.org

The correct citation for this book is

Gabbard GO (ed.): *Countertransference Issues in Psychiatric Treatment* (Review of Psychiatry Series; Oldham JM and Riba MB, series eds.). Washington, DC, American Psychiatric Press, 1999

Library of Congress Cataloging-in-Publication Data
Countertransference issues in psychiatric treatment / edited by Glen O. Gabbard
p. cm. — (Review of psychiatry series ; v. 18, no. 1)
Includes bibliographical references and index.
ISBN 0-88048-959-6 (alk. paper)
1. Countertransference (Psychology). 2. Psychoanalysis. 3. Psychotherapist and patient. I. Gabbard, Glen O. II. Series
[DNLM: 1. Countertransference (Psychology). 2. Psychoanalytic Therapy. WM 62 C8554 1999]
RC489.C68C685 1999
616.89'17—dc21
DNLM/DLC
for Library of Congress 99-10446
CIP

British Library Cataloguing in Publication Data
A CIP record is available from the British Library.

Contents

Contributors

Glen O. Gabbard, M.D. Callaway Distinguished Professor, The Menninger Clinic; Director and Training and Supervising Analyst, Topeka Institute for Psychoanalysis; Clinical Professor of Psychiatry, University of Kansas School of Medicine, Wichita, Kansas

Marcia Kraft Goin, M.D. Clinical Professor of Psychiatry and the Behavioral Sciences, Department of Psychiatry, University of Southern California School of Medicine, Los Angeles, California

Brian Kelly, B.Med., Ph.D., F.R.A.N.Z.C.P. Associate Professor, Department of Psychiatry, University of Queensland; Director, Consultation-Liaison Psychiatry, Princess Alexandra Hospital and District Health Service and Mater Misericordiae Hospital, Brisbane, Queensland, Australia

John R. Lion, M.D. Clinical Professor of Psychiatry, University of Maryland School of Medicine, Baltimore, Maryland

John T. Maltsberger, M.D. Associate Clinical Professor of Psychiatry, Harvard Medical School; Attending Psychiatrist, McLean Hospital, Belmont, Massachusetts; Clinical Associate in Psychiatry, Massachusetts General Hospital, Boston, Massachusetts

John M. Oldham, M.D. Director, New York State Psychiatric Institute; Dollard Professor and Vice Chairman, Department of Psychiatry, Columbia University College of Physicians and Surgeons, New York, New York

Michelle B. Riba, M.D. Clinical Associate Professor of Psychiatry and Associate Chair for Education and Academic Affairs, Department of Psychiatry, University of Michigan Health System, Ann Arbor, Michigan

Francis T. Varghese, M.B.B.S., F.R.A.N.Z.C.P. Associate Professor, Department of Psychiatry, University of Queensland; Chair, Division of Mental Health, Princess Alexandra Hospital and District Health Service, Brisbane, Queensland, Australia

Introduction to the Review of Psychiatry Series

John M. Oldham, M.D., and
Michelle B. Riba, M.D., Series Editors

As this century and millennium come to a close, it seems a universal impulse to pause and "take stock." Any time is a good time to do this, of course, but the big round number 2000 just over the horizon seems a special one. It turns out to be, in our opinion, quite a good time for the field of psychiatry. Although a great deal more work lies ahead, we have made substantial progress in the fight for parity, with stronger partnerships having been built among clinicians, patients, families, and advocates. We are hopefully past the most extreme swing of the pendulum of managed care overcontrol, with a new, quite strong professional voice emerging to articulate and define evidence-based practice guidelines and best practices and to set performance standards and develop quality and outcome indicators for good clinical care.

The explosion of knowledge in neuroscience, meanwhile, only accelerates, with its accompanying breathtaking advances in technology. As more is learned about the circuitry of the brain, we obtain a clearer understanding of neurodevelopment gone awry in vulnerable populations such as those at risk to develop schizophrenia. But as we learn more about the brain's "hard-wiring," an entire frontier of information is unfolding, demonstrating an unprecedented plasticity of the brain. In turn, the sensitive, bidirectional interplay between biology and the environment becomes the name of the game.

In the context of these and many other features of our present landscape, we have chosen for this year's Annual Review a sampling of the latest knowledge and thinking from clinical practice and from the laboratory: 1) countertransference issues in psychiatric treatment, 2) disruptive behavior disorders in children and adolescents, 3) gender differences in mood and anxiety disorders,

4) masculinity and sexuality, and 5) molecular biology of schizophrenia.

We are grateful to our section editors and our authors, who worked hard and successfully to produce the text material. As well, we are indebted to Carol Nadelson, M.D., Claire Reinburg, Pamela Harley, Ron McMillen, and the entire American Psychiatric Press, Inc., staff. And the entire project would not have been possible without the steady help of Sam McGowan and Linda Gacioch.

Foreword

Glen O. Gabbard, M.D.

In a survey of private practitioners and academic psychiatrists, Langsley and Yager (1988) found that the second most highly regarded skill in psychiatry was the ability to "recognize countertransference problems and personal idiosyncrasies as they influence interactions with patients and be able to deal with them constructively" (p. 471). Indeed, one of the unique aspects of psychiatry is that we recognize the continuing influence of our own personal characteristics on the diagnostic and treatment processes we are conducting with our patients. Postmodernist thinking has spread even to science, within which investigators now acknowledge by a broad consensus that what is observed by the scientist is never entirely uncontaminated by the scientist's biases and subjectivity.

Nevertheless, a concept of considerable value like countertransference is somewhat beleaguered these days in an era in which "quick fixes" are encouraged by a managed care system driven by economic values. There is less time for reflection about what is transpiring between doctor and patient and little emphasis placed on the meanings of the interaction. An overarching principle of psychodynamic psychiatry is that we doctors have much in common with the patients we treat (Gabbard 1994). In other words, the psychological mechanisms we observe in pathological states are merely extensions of principles involved in normal developmental functioning. Just as our patients bring a set of transferences to every interaction, we psychiatrists bring our own set of countertransferences that are shaped by the patient's individual characteristics and the interaction itself. There are no interactions in psychiatry that are entirely free of transference-countertransference dynamics.

This book, part of Volume 18 of the Review of Psychiatry series, is designed to restore countertransference's much deserved role as a highly valued conceptual framework for understanding the psychiatrist's contribution to the diagnosis and treatment of the patient. One resident told me not long ago that his inpatient supervisor informed him that "psychodynamics are relevant to outpatients, not to inpatients." In fact, psychodynamic concepts are relevant to every activity that the psychiatrist does, and the chapters in this book recognize that broad application of the concept. One does not have to practice long-term intensive psychoanalytic psychotherapy to observe transference or countertransference.

In the opening chapter, I try to set the stage for what follows by updating the reader with a review of the cutting edge of psychoanalytic theory that involves projective identification, role-responsiveness, countertransference enactments, and subjectivity. I point out that there is an emerging common ground among a variety of different theoretical perspectives within psychoanalysis. In brief, most of the major theories point to countertransference as a jointly created phenomenon involving feelings *induced* by the patient working in tandem with the preexisting self and object representations that the clinician brings to the encounter. I also touch on some of the current controversies about countertransference in terms of technique. When does the psychotherapist disclose countertransference feelings as a constructive means of deepening the process and the understanding of the patient? Also, what mental processes are involved in the containment of powerful feelings generated by the patient?

In the second chapter, Maltsberger extends his classic paper on countertransference hate in treating suicidal patients (Maltsberger and Buie 1973) by elaborating on the common difficulties encountered in the psychotherapy of suicidal patients with borderline personality disorder. With vivid clinical examples, he shows how the therapist is inevitably drawn into the patient's internal world. The necessary empathic connection for good psychotherapy makes the clinician vulnerable to a kind of coercive bondage through projective identification. Narcissistic rage in the clinician may be stimulated, and a variety of defensive maneuvers, including reaction formation and rationalization, can result in highly malignant acting out in an effort to try to keep fantasies of malice out of the clinician's mind. Maltsberger also provides some valuable guidance on how the patient may try to recruit the therapist's permission to go ahead with suicide, through subtle means of presuicidal communications. Maltsberger emphasizes how therapists may share some of the same underlying issues around abandonment that are often attributed to borderline patients.

In the third chapter, Goin examines how countertransference themes apply in the practice of general psychiatry. The same psychodynamic issues relevant to psychotherapy, such as countertransference, transference, and resistance, can also be found in the practice of prescribing medication. Specific types of countertransference difficulties arise when the treatment is split between a pharmacotherapist and a psychotherapist, as it so often is under managed care arrangements in the current health care environment. Similarly, consultation-liaison psychiatry allows the psychiatrist the opportunity to get in touch with the countertransference engendered in hospital staff, who are not necessarily psychiatrically trained. Even in the psychiatric inpatient unit in extremely brief hospitalizations, there are significant patterns of transference and countertransference among hospital staff that reflect a re-creation of the patient's internal object world in the milieu of the unit.

Lion, in his contribution, looks at one of the most difficult categories of patients whom psychiatrists encounter: those with antisocial personality disorder. These patients may pretend to be interested in treatment while secretly "conning" the clinician. They may exploit the treatment for their own purposes, such as getting out of jail. Or they may frighten the clinician by threatening violence. A unique set of countertransference responses is involved in working with these patients, and Lion discusses these responses with considerable insight and a great deal of clinical wisdom. He also explores how the gender of the patient and the nature of the crime influence the clinician's reactions, especially in the context of forensic settings, where countertransferences may occur that are not typically encountered in ordinary clinical settings.

In 1995 the Parliament of the Northern Territory in Australia made it legal for a doctor to give a lethal injection to a patient suffering from terminal illness at that patient's request. The law was later overturned by the Australian Federal Parliament. In the last chapter of this book, Varghese and Kelly bring a unique perspective from "Down Under" to their discussion of physician-assisted suicide. Although much is made of a "rational" decision to assist in ending the life of a person with a terminal illness, the authors point out that those decisions made by medical professionals, including psychiatrists, can never be entirely free of what we would broadly call countertransference issues. The doctor's own anxiety in the face of death, and even the hatred of the patient who does not want treatment or will not allow the doctor to be helpful, can influence a supposedly scientific or "rational" decision. Although we would rather not think about it, the clinician's unconscious wish to kill may lie behind some cases of physician-assisted suicide.

References

Gabbard GO: Psychodynamic Psychiatry in Clinical Practice: The DSM-IV Edition. Washington, DC, American Psychiatric Press, 1994

Langsley DG, Yager J: The definition of a psychiatrist: eight years later. Am J Psychiatry 145:469–475, 1988

Maltsberger JT, Buie DH: Countertransference hate in the treatment of suicidal patients. Arch Gen Psychiatry 30:625–633, 1973

Chapter 1

An Overview of Countertransference: Theory and Technique

Glen O. Gabbard, M.D.

Because the concept of countertransference grows out of the psychoanalytic literature, it may come as a surprise to many to learn that Freud had remarkably little to say about the subject. The notion first appeared in his writings in 1910: "We have become aware of the 'counter-transference,' which arises in [the physician] as a result of the patient's influence on his unconscious feelings . . ." (Freud 1910/1957, p. 144). Freud suggested that the analyst "begin his activity with a self-analysis and continually carry it deeper while he is making his observations on his patients" (p. 145).

In Freud's view, countertransference is essentially an obstacle to be overcome. The doctor unconsciously experiences the patient as someone from the doctor's past. In this regard, the countertransference could be conceptualized as the analyst's transference to the patient. This Freudian view is commonly referred to as the *narrow* perspective, and it is still espoused by some modern classical analysts (e.g., Brenner 1982).

Freud's relative silence on the subject of countertransference does not necessarily reflect his lack of interest in the topic. Rather, he felt it was indiscreet to speak so forthrightly about the analyst's vulnerability, especially in light of his concern that his young science might be jeopardized by such open discussions. In a December 31, 1911, letter to Carl Jung, Freud made his position clear on this matter:

> Frau C—— has told me all sorts of things about you and Pfister, if you can call the hints she drops "telling." I gather that neither of

> you has yet acquired the necessary objectivity in your practice, that you still get involved, giving a good deal of yourselves and expecting the patient to give something in return. Permit me, speaking as the venerable old master, to say that this technique is invariably ill-advised and that it is best to remain reserved and purely receptive. We must never let our poor neurotics drive us crazy. I believe an article on "counter-transference" is sorely needed; of course we could not publish it, we should have to circulate copies among ourselves. (McGuire 1974, pp. 475–476)

Freud's cautionary note was taken seriously for several decades, but it has largely gone unheeded in contemporary discourse on psychoanalysis and psychotherapy. Discussions of clinical process today typically include accounts of the analyst's or therapist's reactions to the patient, often with considerable candor, to underscore the idea that there are two persons in the consulting room and that each affects the other. Open acknowledgment of countertransference is in keeping with a conceptual shift from the view that psychoanalysis is a one-person psychology focused on the intrapsychic world of the patient to a broad consensus that it involves both a one-person and a two-person perspective. This shift is just as relevant to intensive psychotherapy, and the discussion of countertransference in this chapter applies to both analysis and therapy. It also reflects a different understanding of countertransference that largely originated from British contributions.

Beginning with Paula Heimann's classic 1950 contribution, countertransference took on a much broader connotation. Heimann suggested that the analyst's total emotional response to the patient is not simply an obstacle or hindrance based on the analyst's own past, but an important tool in understanding the patient's unconscious. This view is often referred to as the *broad* or *totalistic* perspective on countertransference. It should be clarified, however, that even though Heimann regarded the countertransference as useful information, she opposed the therapist's communicating his or her feelings to the patient.

Writing at about the same time, D. W. Winnicott (1949) also argued for the usefulness of countertransference. He felt that in some cases there was an *objective* form of countertransference in which the therapist reacted to the patient in the same way that everyone else did. For example, certain patients would be so provocative and contemptuous that everyone with whom they came into contact, including the therapist, would respond by hating them. In Winnicott's view, this hateful reaction had much less to do with the therapist's own personal past or his or her intrapsychic conflicts and much more to do with the patient's behavior and need to evoke specific reactions in others.

Today clinicians of all persuasions generally accept the idea that countertransference can be a useful source of information about the patient (Abend 1989; Gabbard 1995). At the same time, the therapist's own subjectivity is involved in the way the patient's behavior is experienced. Hence, there is a movement in the direction of regarding countertransference as a *jointly created* phenomenon that involves contributions from both patient and clinician. The patient draws the therapist into playing a role that reflects the patient's internal world, but the specific dimensions of that role are colored by the therapist's own personality (Gabbard 1995). This contemporary understanding can best be illustrated by an examination of several key concepts in the current psychoanalytic literature: projective identification, role-responsiveness, countertransference enactment, and relational/constructivist theories.

Key Concepts in Countertransference

Projective Identification

The term *projective identification* has now become commonplace in American psychiatry, largely because of its usefulness in clinical work with patients who have severe personality disorders (Gabbard and Wilkinson 1994; Kernberg 1975). Nevertheless, the term is used in different ways by different clinicians and theoreticians, and thus one cannot be certain of the specific meaning that applies to the term in any given instance.

Melanie Klein originated the term in her 1946 paper "Notes on Some Schizoid Mechanisms" (Klein 1946/1975). Although the concept was not the cornerstone of the paper, much has been made of Klein's use of the term by subsequent commentators. For the most part, British analysts understand her use of the term as essentially a fantasy in which part of the patient's self is split off and projected into the therapist without necessarily altering the way the therapist feels or behaves. In essence, the entire process is an intrapsychic one (Segal 1964; Spillius 1992). If the analyst was influenced by the patient's behavior, Klein regarded it as a reflection of countertransference in the narrow sense and saw it as a sign that the analyst required further analysis. Klein disagreed with Heimann's broadened perspective because she felt it might facilitate the blaming of patients for the analyst's countertransference problems.

On the other hand, some American analysts, especially Ogden (1979, 1982, 1994), proposed a different reading of Klein's work. Ogden pointed out that Klein preferred the preposition *into* rather than *onto* when describing the fate of projected contents. This usage reflected the possibility of an interpersonal aspect of projective identification. Further evidence of this conceptualization was the way Klein used the term in a subsequent paper, "On Identification," published in 1955 (Klein 1955/1975). This contribution focused on a science fiction novella in which the protagonist projected himself into others and took them over from the inside. Ogden suggested that the usage of projective identification in this instance of applied psychoanalysis clearly implied that the target of the projection is ultimately transformed by the process.

Several of Klein's British colleagues also suggested that there was an interpersonal dimension to the projective identification mechanism (Bion 1955; Money-Kyrle 1956; Rosenfeld 1952). Bion, in particular, was instrumental in influencing Ogden and other American analysts by linking projective identification with his container-contained model of infant-mother and patient-analyst interaction (Bion 1957/1967, 1958/1967, 1959/1967, 1962a/1967, 1962b/1967, 1970). In his view, the infant handles intolerable affects by disavowing them and projecting them into the mother. The mother then contains them and "detoxifies" them before they are reinternalized by the infant, who can then manage them more fully through identification with the mother's containment of them. Bion left no doubt that this process was not simply an unconscious fantasy of the infant but an explicitly interpersonal interaction between the two parties. Similarly, in the therapeutic situation, the patient would behave in such a way that the therapist felt coerced into playing a role in the patient's fantasy.

Ogden (1979, 1982) later elaborated on the work of Bion by describing three aspects of projective identification: 1) an aspect of the self (usually a self or object representation connected with an affect) is projectively disavowed by the patient's unconsciously placing it in the therapist or analyst; 2) the patient exerts interpersonal pressure that coerces the therapist to experience or unconsciously identify with that which has been projected; and 3) the recipient of the projection in the therapeutic situation processes and contains the projected contents, and this leads to reintrojection by the patient in modified form. Ogden (1992) later stressed that these aspects should not be understood as occurring in a linear sequence of steps. Instead, he felt there was a dialectic created in which the patient and therapist enter into a relationship in which they are simultaneously separate but also "at one" with each other. Each has a unique subjectivity that contributes to the unique transference-countertransference dimensions within the dyad. In this regard, projective identification is conceptualized as not only a defense mechanism but also a means of communication from patient to analyst in a specific object.

A clinical example will illustrate the process. A patient says to the therapist, "You hate me, and I know it." The therapist, taken by surprise, responds by asking, "What makes you say that?" The patient becomes angry and glowers at the therapist: "Don't act like you don't know what I'm talking about!" The therapist protests: "But I don't!" The patient shouts at the therapist: "You liar! You know exactly what I mean!" At this point the therapist, feeling enraged, says, "I don't appreciate being called a liar!" The patient appears triumphant and says, "You see? I'm right! You *do* hate me. Your face is red, and your eyes are filled with hate!" In this vignette, the patient projects a hating internal object into the therapist. She then behaves in such an infuriating manner that she coerces the therapist to take on the characteristics of the "bad object." His obvious anger is interpreted by her as confirmation that he hates her.

The analyst's or therapist's reactions to what has been projected by the patient are an area of some controversy within psychoanalytic theory and technique. Racker (1968) divided the analyst's reactions into concordant and complementary countertransferences. The former involves an empathic link between the analyst and patient; in other words, the analyst identifies with a self representation within the patient. Complementary countertransferences involve the analyst's identification with an internal object representation of the patient, which Racker regarded as an instance in which the analyst's own conflicts are activated by the patient's projections.

Grinberg (1979) made a further distinction in terms of the analyst's response when he coined the term *projective counteridentification.* In his view, Racker's complementary countertransference reaction should also be regarded as a function of the patient's projection corresponding with certain aspects of the analyst's own unconscious conflicts. On the other hand, in projective counteridentification, Grinberg suggested, the analyst introjects an affective state associated with the patient's object representation that comes almost entirely from the patient. Most contemporary thinkers would consider Grinberg's view an extreme one.

Most contemporary Kleinians now accept the notion that the therapist's countertransference may reflect the patient's attempt to evoke feelings in the therapist that the patient cannot tolerate. Joseph (1989), for example, noted that patients often attempt to "nudge" the analyst to behave in a manner that corresponds to what the patient is projecting. When analysts respond in an attenuated way to what they are having evoked in them by the patient, they become consciously aware of the patient's internal world and are able to help the patient understand it through interpretation. Spillius (1992) argues that the analyst is inevitably influenced to some degree by whatever the patient is projecting. On the other hand, she also stresses that there is a virtually universal consensus that the patient can never be blamed for all the feelings experienced by the therapist. There is an ever-present risk that therapists may confuse their own feelings with those of the patient. Hence, part of the analyst's or therapist's task is to process what is transpiring in the dyad in such a way that his or her own feelings are differentiated from those originating in the patient.

A common thread in these contributions is that mental contents are not mystically transported from patient to clinician. Rather, interpersonal pressure is applied by specific patient behaviors that evoke specific clinician responses. These coercive pressures from the patient have an obligatory quality to them that makes them extremely difficult to resist. Although it may feel as if an alien force has taken over the recipient of the projection, in actuality what has happened is that an aspect of the recipient's internal world has been activated by the behavior of the projector (Gabbard 1995). The analyst's or therapist's usual sense of a familiar, continuous self is disrupted by his or her own repressed self or object representations emerging in response to the patient's interpersonal pressure. In this regard the process of projective identification requires a "hook" in the recipient of the projection to make it stick. Thus, some clinicians will be a better "fit" than others with the patient's projections.

Of course, this formulation also raises the possibility that the countertransference jointly created will vary from one clinician to the next. Feldman (1997), another contemporary Kleinian who has given a good deal of thought to projective identification, made the following observation: "The phantasies of archaic object relationships must inevitably resonate with the analyst's own unconscious needs and anxieties. If these relate too closely to areas of conflict that remain largely unresolved, there are dangers that the analyst will be driven into forms of enactment that either gratify some mutual needs or defend him against such gratification" (p. 239). Here Feldman emphasizes that what is projected is actually a fantasied object relationship rather than simply a part of the patient. Moreover, the involvement of the object as a recipient of the projection is a key characteristic of the projective identification process. He further stresses that although the patient's projections are designed to reduce the discrepancy between the fantasied object relationship and the actual experience of the analytic situation, the analyst must work diligently to attempt to extricate himself or herself from the pressure to enact the object relationship and recover the capacity for reflective thought. The more the therapist can attend to the discrepancy between the reality of the therapeutic situation and the patient's internal pressure to transform the therapist into a transference object, the more the therapist can create a space to examine the interaction in collaboration with the patient.

For example, patients with borderline personality disorder who have a history of childhood trauma may unconsciously re-create the abusive relationship from the past by behaving contemptuously toward the therapist. If the therapist resists the transformation into the bad object role, the patient may simply escalate the behavior and become more contemptuous or increase specific kinds of acting-out behavior to attempt to get a rise out of the therapist. On the other hand, if the therapist "gives in" and allows transformation into the patient's bad object, the capacity to be therapeutic may be destroyed. Hence, the therapist must strive for a middle ground where there is an attenuated or partial enactment of the bad object role, perhaps by becoming irritated with the patient, but also the preservation of the capacity for reflective thought so that the interaction can be explored with the patient. The therapist might say to the patient, for example: "I sense that it is important for you to irritate me by regarding me with such contempt, but I also think the two of us need to try to understand what is so compelling about getting under my skin in this way."

Role-Responsiveness

Joseph Sandler originated the concept of *role-responsiveness* in a classic 1976 paper. A contemporary Freudian rather than a Kleinian, Sandler nonetheless described a process closely related to the contemporary view of projective identification: "Very often the irrational response of the analyst, which his professional conscience leads him to see entirely as a blind spot of his own, may sometimes be usefully regarded as a compromise-formation between his own tendencies and *his reflexive acceptance of the role which the patient is forcing on him*" (1976, p. 46). In this formulation, Sandler regarded the patient as unconsciously actualizing an internalized object relationship in the transference with the therapist. The therapist then plays a role derived from the patient's intrapsychic world. Spillius (1992) emphasizes that Sandler's view is essentially the same as Joseph's observation that the patient unconsciously induces feelings in the analyst and then nudges the analyst into acting in a manner that is in accord with the projection.

Sandler (1993), in a subsequent paper, distinguishes role-responsiveness from a process of *primary identification.* He describes the latter as an automatic mirroring process that underlies empathy. Expressing concern that there is a state that is induced by the patient, Sandler stresses that we cannot assume a one-to-one correspondence between what goes on in the analyst and what goes on in the patient.

In Sandler's view, to warrant the label "projective identification," the analyst's emotional reaction to the patient's behavior must be the result of an unconscious intent in the patient to evoke such a reaction in the analyst. The therapist uses projective identification as a defensive process that has two essential steps: 1) intrapsychic projection of a split-off and unwanted aspect of a self representation into an object representation and 2) externalization of the object representation via an actualization process in which the analyst is pressured through verbal and nonverbal maneuvers, largely unconscious, to play a particular role with the patient.

Countertransference Enactment

Whereas the literature on projective identification and role-responsiveness has largely emanated from the United Kingdom, most of the contributions on *countertransference enactment* have been written by American analysts associated with an ego psychological perspective (Chused 1991; Jacobs 1986; McLaughlin 1991). Enactment is often used in the broad sense by these authors to indicate subtle instances of interlocking transference-countertransference dimensions that operate outside the therapist's conscious awareness. Nonverbal correlates, such as tensing of muscles, changes in breathing, or shifts in body posture, are often used as illustrations. In addition, much of the writing from this perspective focuses to a large extent on the narrow aspects of countertransference—that is, experiences from the analyst's past that are revived in the interaction with the patient.

Nonetheless, Chused's useful definition of countertransference enactment is closely linked to projective identification: "Enactments occur when an attempt to actualize the transference fantasy elicits a countertransference reaction" (Chused 1991, p. 629). Roughton (1993) notes the similarity between countertransference enactment and projective identification. However, he asserts that enactments may involve putting an experience into behavior. Actualization, on the other hand, is viewed as involving a subtle form of manipulation that induces the analyst to behave or speak in a way that resembles the particular role that the analysand hopes to impose on the analyst. Roughton would call this an enactment that has an actualizing effect. He stresses that this point of view is virtually identical with Sandler's role-responsiveness and Ogden's understanding of projective identification.

Although the ego psychologists writing about countertransference enactment would agree that the analyst is being pressured to become the transference object of the patient, they would stress a greater contribution from the analyst's unconscious conflicts than is typical of those writing from a Kleinian perspective. However, this is simply a difference in emphasis rather than in substance. Another difference between enactment and projective identification is that enactment by definition implies an action. Some would argue that it is at least theoretically possible for projective identification to induce a countertransference feeling without that feeling's being carried into action. This distinction becomes rather tenuous, though, if one includes subtle shifts in body posture or tone of voice as actions.

Relational/Constructivist Theories

Both relational and constructivist theories emphasize the mutuality of the therapeutic relationship. Two subjectivities are present and are mutually influencing each other. Central to the constructivist perspective is the idea that enactments are going on continuously in both directions, and therapists must continually monitor themselves to understand how they might be unconsciously participating in an internal scenario scripted by the patient (Gill 1991; Hoffman 1992). These theorists also stress that the analyst's actual behavior influences the patient's transference to the analyst. Hence, both transference and countertransference are jointly constructed on the basis of the mutual influence of the two parties. Also, within this point of view, transference and countertransference are inextricably linked.

A more radical aspect of constructivist thought is that countertransference is not simply a reaction to the patient. To view countertransference as only reactive risks polarizing the analyst's role as initiator and the analyst's role as reactor. Hoffman (1991) advocates a model in which "responsiveness is understood to be simultaneously self-expressive, just as self-expressive initiative is understood to be simultaneously responsive to the other person in the interaction" (p. 98).

Relational thinkers, like constructivists, point out that our traditional model of transference-countertransference may understate the analyst's responsibility for initiating a sequence of interactional events. Aron (1995) has even suggested that it may be impossible to sort out who initiated a particular sequence of interaction and that therefore the distinction between countertransference and subjectivity is not particularly useful.

Implied in this model is an increased vulnerability in the analyst. The analyst's countertransference, as well as the real characteristics of the analyst, is constantly exposed to the patient. The patient may accurately tune in to aspects of the analyst's feelings, and exploration of the patient's perception of the analyst is a critical part of the technique. Hence, relational and constructivist thinkers would encourage the patient to elaborate on his or her fantasies about the analyst's experience (Aron 1995; Hoffman 1983).

Relational theorists such as Mitchell (1988, 1993), Aron (1995), Hirsch (1993, 1994), and Tansey (1994) have arrived at conclusions about the inevitability and usefulness of countertransference enactments that are largely in keeping with the views of some American ego psychologists and of many Kleinians. Mitchell (1988) pointed out how his own views resemble those of Sandler and Gill:

> The analyst is regarded as, at least to some degree, embedded within the analysand's relational matrix. There is no way for the analyst to avoid his assigned roles and configurations within the analysand's relational world. The analyst's experience is necessarily shaped by the analysand's relational structure; he plays assigned roles even if he desperately tries to stand outside the patient's system and play no role at all." (p. 292)

Consensus and Controversy

The overview presented in the foregoing section suggests that theorists from diverse persuasions have converged on the idea that, to some extent, countertransference is a joint creation involving contributions from both clinician and patient. The relative emphasis given to each of these contributions may vary with the theory, but there is a remarkable degree of agreement that what the patient projects onto the clinician and what the clinician brings to the situation are both relevant to the end result of countertransference. There is also widespread agreement that the patient will inevitably attempt to transform the therapist into a transference object. The therapist must then work diligently to find a way out of the transference-countertransference enactment or projected role that the patient thrusts on him or her.

The image of the analyst or therapist as a blank screen maintaining complete neutrality and anonymity is no longer a viable concept. Countertransference is inevitable and useful as part of an exploration involving two spontaneous and responsive individuals engaged in an intense and emotionally taxing interaction. By acknowledging the full partnership of the two parties, one is acknowledging the greater exposure of the therapist to scrutiny by the patient and the ever-present threat of countertransferential self-protectiveness (Greenberg 1991).

Another risk is that the clinician will mistake mutuality for symmetry (Aron 1995). Although there are two parties engaged in a relationship, one is paying the other a fee for a professional service. One does not belong to a professional organization that sets and enforces ethical standards, whereas the other does. One is the recipient of help from the other. Hence, the need for professional boundaries must be remembered in an era in which the spontaneous and emotional involvement of the clinician is acknowledged and taken for granted (Gabbard and Lester 1995).

Role of Countertransference Enactments

One of the major controversies in the area of countertransference is whether or not the enactments are useful to the process. Although most of the contributors to this dialogue acknowledge the inevitability of countertransference enactments, they have different views about whether enactments are therapeutic. Chused (1991), for example, has stressed that the value for the treatment is not in the enactment itself but rather in the examination and eventual understanding of the enactment. Renik (1993) suggests that awareness of countertransference can emerge only after a countertransference enactment has occurred. The enactment itself, in his view, may have therapeutic value, a view shared by Eagle (1993). Jacobs (1993) takes a middle course in which he regards experience and insight operating together. Hence, the enactment itself and the examination of it cannot be separated from each other in terms of the therapeutic action in psychoanalytic treatment.

In the Menninger Treatment Intervention Project (Horwitz et al. 1996), audiotaped transcripts of psychotherapy with patients with borderline personality disorder were studied by a team of researchers. One of the findings was that partial transference gratifications produced by countertransference enactments seemed to have therapeutic value even when they were not analyzed fully. For example, in one case studied by the investigators, a patient repeatedly threatened to quit the therapy. The therapist responded by verbally pursuing the patient and insisting that he felt she was not ready to terminate. Although one could argue that he was at least partially gratifying her transference wish to be pursued and asked to continue therapy, clearly the patient experienced his countertransference enactment as a sign that he cared about her and was engaged in trying to help her find a way to continue in treatment. The countertransference enactment was also suffused with the conviction that the patient was treatable and could be helped by the process. The patient ultimately stayed for approximately 2 years of therapy and was rated by independent judges as considerably improved.

In this clinical situation the therapist was not aware of acting on countertransference. Rather, he felt he was doing what was in the patient's best interest. In this context it is important to emphasize that countertransference as originally defined is unconscious, at least initially, before the enactments and self-observational capacities of the clinician begin to make the feelings available to conscious awareness. Often the therapist struggles for considerable periods of time with multifaceted affective experiences or behaviors that cannot be defined and articulated. Much of the therapist's self-analytic work may be directed to understanding the meaning of those behaviors or affective states.

Therapist Self-Disclosure

Another controversy related to countertransference entails how to translate the therapist's feelings into useful interventions with the patient. In recent years, self-disclosure of countertransference feelings has become much more of an acceptable part of psychotherapeutic technique. Indeed, with the demise of the blank-screen stereotype, virtually all clinicians acknowledge that they make self-disclosures of various types on an ongoing basis. Therapists decorate their offices in ways that reflect their subjectivity. The way they dress, their manner of speech, and their nonverbal communications convey all kinds of information about them. Indeed, they disclose something about themselves whenever they choose to comment on a particular aspect of what the patient is saying.

However, these inadvertent self-disclosures are not the same as specific technical interventions designed to allow one to use the countertransference constructively. Unfortunately, it is an enormous challenge to try to create a set of technical guidelines on when self-disclosure is useful and when it is not. Perhaps the best one can say is that in *some* treatments, in *some* situations, with *some* patients, and about *some* feelings, self-disclosures may be constructive. Another general guideline is that there is merit in *restraint* about revealing one's personal struggles. It is not a good or ethical use of the patient's time or money to burden the patient with the therapist's emotional problems.

Renik (1995) has argued that the therapist's feelings in some cases are apparent to the patient and to deny them is disingenuous. If, for example, the patient has angered the therapist and the therapist is visibly upset, it may be useful to corroborate the patient's perception. If the patient says, "Are you angry?," the therapist might say, "I think you're accurately picking up some of my feelings, and I hope we can understand what is happening here to make me angry. It may be useful for the treatment if we can make some connections between the interaction here and what happens with others outside of here."

This kind of clinical honesty in the here and now can be particularly helpful for severely disturbed patients, such as those with borderline personality disorder, who have a difficult time understanding the impact they have on others (Gabbard and Wilkinson 1994). On the other hand, disclosures of certain specific countertransference feelings may be deeply disquieting to patients. Disclosure of sexual feelings for a patient, even if the patient demands to know the therapist's feelings, may come perilously close to feeling like an incest taboo has been broken (Gabbard 1994, 1996; Gabbard and Lester 1995). In our society, disclosure of sexual feelings implies an action, and the patient-therapist relationship does not exist outside that culture. The patient may feel that the therapist is dangerously out of control and may flee the treatment. No matter how well intentioned such disclosures may be, the therapist has no idea of the impact the disclosures will ultimately have on the patient.

Nor can therapists know with any certainty what their own unconscious agenda is when they decide to self-disclose. A profession of love, for example, may unconsciously be masking anger toward the patient. Whatever is disclosed may fail to capture the complexity of the therapist's experience as well. Greenberg

(1995) noted, "There are always multiple perspectives on the participation of each party. This means that whatever is revealed is simply one person's understanding in a given moment—never . . . the last word on the subject. . . . I am not necessarily in a privileged position to know, much less to reveal, everything that I think or feel" (p. 197). Anything that the therapist reveals is likely to conceal other feelings. Hence, it is probably best to err on the side of restraint and thoughtfulness when contemplating self-disclosures of countertransference feelings.

Therapists may often feel cornered into self-disclosure, but in such situations the therapist still has a variety of options other than dishonest denial of certain feelings or forced disclosure. For example, if a patient demands to know whether the therapist finds him or her sexually attractive, the therapist may proceed in any number of ways:

1. Inquire why at this particular time and on this particular day that information has become so compelling.
2. Point out how others have answered that question for the patient but how the answer does not seem to help the patient's fundamental problem with self-esteem.
3. Address the patient's insistence and coerciveness and point to how they may undermine the patient's getting the kind of answers that he or she wants.
4. Disclose the personal dilemma in which the patient is placing the therapist. The therapist might, for example, respond: "You place me in a dilemma when you demand to know whether I find you sexually attractive. Either way I answer the question could lead to significant problems for the therapy. If I say that I do not find you attractive, you may feel devastated. If I say that I do, you may feel that the therapy is not as safe a place as you previously thought."

The main point in regard to these situations is that the therapist has considerable latitude. In general, when the therapist is not feeling comfortable about answering a specific question involving countertransference feelings, the therapist might be better off examining the process than going directly to the content of the question. Moreover, the therapist's discomfort with disclosing certain feelings is a legitimate reason not to do so.

Containment of Countertransference Feelings

Direct self-disclosure of countertransference feelings is often contrasted with containment of those feelings that ultimately lead to interpretation. In the reality of clinical practice, containment and self-disclosure are by no means mutually exclusive and often work together synergistically. In other words, containing and processing countertransference feelings may facilitate a more constructive disclosure of how the therapist is feeling and why. Nevertheless, for purposes of this discussion, they will be considered separately.

In discussions of the therapeutic action of psychotherapy and psychoanalysis, containing and tolerating the countertransference feelings are often viewed as mutative in and of themselves (Carpy 1989). By observing the therapist's capacity to handle affects that are regarded as intolerable, the patient comes to realize that the feelings are not as unmanageable as previously thought. The patient may then reintroject the feelings and the self and object representations associated with those feelings and find that they may be more easily tolerated.

The term *containment* is often used interchangeably with *holding*; both concepts involve a host of interrelated internal processes. Containment is sometimes viewed incorrectly as simply masochistic endurance of the unpleasant behavior of a difficult patient. However, it is actually an active process that involves a set of internal activities that can be subdivided into several categories (Gabbard and Wilkinson 1994).

Diagnosis of the Patient's Internal Object Relations

The feelings stirred in the clinician are likely to reflect aspects of the patient's internal world. One of the advantages of containing feelings and postponing interpretation of what is transpiring between patient and therapist is that the therapist has the opportunity to gain a greater understanding of how the patient's internal world is influencing the therapist. Bion (1974) spoke about the need to delay interpretive interventions:

> Psycho-analysts must be able to tolerate the differences or the difficulties of the analysand long enough to recognize what they are. If psycho-analysts are to be able to interpret what the analysand says, they must have a great capacity for tolerating their analysand's statements without rushing to the conclusion that they know the interpretations. (p. 72)

The therapist may be pushed and pulled in a variety of directions that seem chaotic at first blush. If the therapist can sit with the feelings for a sufficient period, he or she may ultimately make sense out of the chaos. The therapist may feel an urge to rescue, chide, cajole, flatter, seduce, criticize, or collude with the patient. Over time, certain object relations paradigms become clear, and the therapist can then make interventions that allow the patient to see how recurrent patterns of object relations are being reenacted in the relationship with the therapist.

Restoration of Reflective Functioning

The patient's projective identification tends to collapse the therapist's necessary "play space," where the interaction with the patient can be both experienced and observed at the same time. The optimal state of mind for therapists is the state of double consciousness that Ogden (1982) refers to as *analytic space.* In this frame of mind, the therapist is "sucked in" to the patient's inner world while retaining the capacity to reflect on what is happening and to bring understanding to the situation. It often takes a significant period of time to recognize that an enactment is occurring so that it can then be reflected on.

Self-Analysis and Self-Examination

The term *containment* is often used as though it refers only to the processing and tolerating of the *patient's* feelings. In fact, the therapist is always containing countertransference responses of his or her own at the same time that the patient's feelings are being held. Hence, another function going on during the containment process is the therapist's self-examination and self-analysis of his or her own contributions to the intense feelings generated in the clinician-patient dyad. To avoid the trap of blaming the patient for all of the therapist's countertransference feelings, the therapist needs to scrutinize how the current situation may resemble a past situation. Therapists must make a concerted effort to sort out their contributions from those of the patient.

Clinicians who wish to treat their patients with intensive psychotherapy or psychoanalysis must first have their own personal treatment experience so that they become familiar with the nature of their intrapsychic object relations and their unconscious conflicts. Part of the work of the psychodynamic therapist or psychoanalyst is rigorous self-analysis so as to avoid the potential problem of drawing the patient into one's own unconscious enactments, thus serving one's needs rather than the patient's. In therapeutic dyads in which the feelings are particularly intense, much of the self-analytic work may go on between sessions, when the therapist analyzes dreams relevant to the treatment and free-associates about specific aspects of the interaction with the patient. Is the patient reminiscent of someone from the therapist's past? Does the patient have qualities in common with a key figure in the therapist's current life? Is the interaction with the patient reminiscent of other situations in the therapist's life in which things are conflictual or difficult?

Internal Supervision

Closely allied with self-examination and self-analysis is what Casement (1985) has referred to as "internal supervision." Trial identifications with the patient through empathy are an important part of this internal supervision function. Therapists can then observe what happens when they empathically place themselves in the shoes of the patient and gain a greater understanding of the patient's internal world. Casement suggests that an internal supervision process originates when therapists are in their own treatments. He refers to such a process as "that island of contemplation from which they can observe with their analyst what they were experiencing in the transference" (p. 31). In addition, most therapists make significant identifications with influential supervisors. Often the therapist carries on an internal dialogue with an internal representation of that supervisor to try to understand situations in which the transference-countertransference dimensions are difficult to manage.

Silent Interpretation

In the throes of powerful feelings, the psychotherapist may feel the need to unload negative affect states by prematurely interpreting what the patient is doing to the therapist. Often when such interventions grow out of a pressured and negative affect state, the patient experiences the interpretation as an attack, and this makes it difficult to listen to the meaning of the intervention.

Silent interpretation may be a better alternative as an initial step toward eventual verbal formulation of the therapeutic situation. As part of the diagnosis of the patient's internal object relations and the restoration of reflective functioning, the therapist can begin to formulate silently what is happening in the dyad. An internal narrative can be developed while the therapist waits for the patient to be in a more receptive and reflective state in which the interpretation can be heard and understood.

Verbal Clarification

In keeping with the notion that containment is not simply a silent and painful enduring of emotional abuse from the patient, a variety of useful verbal interventions can be made as part of the containment process. These comments are largely in the nature of clarifications. The therapist may repackage what the patient has said in order to draw together similar themes. For example, when the patient is ventilating anger, the therapist might say, "So it sounds like you've been angry at me for taking vacations at times when you feel you need me most. Have there been other situations in your life when similar feelings have arisen?" Clarifications can be followed by invitations to expand and elaborate on the patient's feelings and perceptions. Excessive silence on the part of the therapist can create considerable difficulties, especially with more severely disturbed patients. They may experience the silence as a lack of engagement or an abandonment. Certain patients also may become increasingly paranoid with excessive silence. Hence, another function of making verbal clarifications is to maintain a connection with the patient that strengthens the therapeutic alliance.

❖

All of these components of containment come together in the actual clinical situation, and they may or may not lead to an interpretation delivered to the patient. As in all psychotherapeutic situations, the therapist must weigh the pros and cons of interpretive versus supportive comments in the context of the patient's strengths and weaknesses at the particular juncture of the therapy.

Conclusion

Countertransference has moved to the very heart of psychoanalytic and psychotherapeutic theory and technique. It has evolved from a narrow conceptualization of the therapist's transference to the patient to a complex and jointly created phenomenon that is pervasive in the treatment process. To a large extent, countertransference is determined by the fit between what the patient projects into the therapist and what preexisting structures are present in the therapist's intrapsychic world. Writings on technique suggest a much greater tolerance for the inevitable partial enactments of countertransference that occur in a treatment process. These enactments provide valuable information about what is being re-created in the psychotherapeutic or psychoanalytic setting. In this regard, therapists must recognize that they will be drawn into various roles in the course of the therapy and that maintaining an artificial aloofness is neither desirable nor helpful. Controversies continue to exist around the therapeutic usefulness of the enactments themselves, versus the retrospective analysis of the enactments, and about the value of direct disclosure of countertransference feelings.

References

Abend SM: Countertransference and technique. Psychoanal Q 48: 374–395, 1989

Aron L: A Meeting of Minds: Mutuality and Psychoanalysis. Hillsdale, NJ, Analytic Press, 1995
Bion WR: Language and the schizophrenic, in New Directions in Psychoanalysis. Edited by Klein M, Heimann P, Money-Kyrle RE. London, Tavistock, 1955, pp 220–239
Bion WR: Differentiation of the psychotic from the non-psychotic personalities. Int J Psychoanal 38:266–275, 1957 (reprinted in Second Thoughts: Selected Papers on Psycho-Analysis. London, Heinemann, 1967, pp 43–64)
Bion WR: On arrogance. Int J Psychoanal 39:144–146, 1958 (reprinted in Second Thoughts: Selected Papers on Psycho-Analysis. London, Heinemann, 1967, pp 86–92)
Bion WR: Attacks on linking. Int J Psychoanal 40:308–315, 1959 (reprinted in Second Thoughts: Selected Papers on Psycho-Analysis. London, Heinemann, 1967, pp 93–100)
Bion WR: Learning From Experience. London, Heinemann, 1962a
Bion WR: The psycho-analytic study of thinking, II: a theory of thinking. Int J Psychoanal 43:306–310, 1962b (reprinted in Second Thoughts: Selected Papers on Psycho-Analysis. London, Heinemann, 1967, pp 110–119)
Bion WR: Attention and Interpretation. London, Tavistock, 1970
Bion WR: Bion's Brazilian Lectures, I. Rio de Janeiro, Imago Editora, 1974
Brenner C: The Mind in Conflict. New York, International Universities Press, 1982
Carpy DV: Tolerating the countertransference: a mutative process. Int J Psychoanal 70:287–294, 1989
Casement P: On Learning From the Patient. London, Tavistock, 1985
Chused JF: The evocative power of enactments. J Am Psychoanal Assoc 39:615–639, 1991
Eagle M: Enactments, transference, and symptomatic cure: a case history. Psychoanalytic Dialogues 3:93–110, 1993
Feldman M: Projective identification: the analyst's involvement. Int J Psychoanal 78:227–241, 1997
Freud S: The future prospects of psycho-analytic therapy (1910), in The Standard Edition of the Complete Psychological Works of Sigmund Freud, Vol 11. Translated and edited by Strachey J. London, Hogarth Press, 1957, pp 139–152
Gabbard GO: Commentary on papers by Tansey, Hirsch, and Davies. Psychoanalytic Dialogues 4:203–213, 1994
Gabbard GO: Countertransference: the emerging common ground. Int J Psychoanal 76:475–485, 1995
Gabbard GO: Love and Hate in the Analytic Setting. Northvale, NJ, Jason Aronson, 1996

Gabbard GO, Lester EP: Boundaries and Boundary Violations in Psychoanalysis. Washington, DC, American Psychiatric Press, 1995

Gabbard GO, Wilkinson SM: Management of Countertransference With Borderline Patients. Washington, DC, American Psychiatric Press, 1994

Gill MM: Indirect suggestion: a response to Oremland's "Interpretation and Interaction," in Interpretation and Interaction: Psychoanalysis or Psychotherapy? Edited by Oremland JD. Hillsdale, NJ, Analytic Press, 1991, pp 137–163

Greenberg JR: Countertransference and reality. Psychoanalytic Dialogues 1:52–73, 1991

Greenberg JR: Self-disclosure: is it psychoanalytic? Contemporary Psychoanalysis 31:193–205, 1995

Grinberg L: Countertransference and projective counteridentification, in Countertransference. Edited by Epstein L, Feiner AH. New York, Jason Aronson, 1979, pp 169–191

Heimann P: On counter-transference. Int J Psychoanal 31:81–84, 1950

Hirsch I: Countertransference enactments and some issues related to external factors in the analyst's life. Psychoanalytic Dialogues 3: 343–366, 1993

Hirsch I: Countertransference love and theoretical model. Psychoanalytic Dialogues 4:171–192, 1994

Hoffman IZ: The patient as interpreter of the analyst's experience. Contemporary Psychoanalysis 19:389–422, 1983

Hoffman IZ: Discussion: Toward a social-constructivist view of the psychoanalytic situation. Psychoanalytic Dialogues 1:74–105, 1991

Hoffman IZ: Some practical implications of a social-constructivist view of the psychoanalytic situation. Psychoanalytic Dialogues 2: 287–304, 1992

Horwitz L, Gabbard GO, Allen JG, et al: Borderline Personality Disorder: Tailoring the Psychotherapy to the Patient. Washington, DC, American Psychiatric Press, 1996

Jacobs TJ: On countertransference enactments. J Am Psychoanal Assoc 34:289–307, 1986

Jacobs TJ: Insight and experience: commentary on Morris Eagle's "Enactments, Transference, and Symptomatic Cure." Psychoanalytic Dialogues 3:123–127, 1993

Joseph B: Psychic Equilibrium and Psychic Change: Selected Papers of Betty Joseph. Edited by Feldman M, Spillius EB. London, Routledge, 1989

Kernberg OF: Borderline Conditions of Pathological Narcissism. New York, Jason Aronson, 1975

Klein M: Notes on some schizoid mechanisms (1946), in Envy and Gratitude and Other Works, 1946–1963. New York, Delacorte Press/Seymour Laurence, 1975, pp 1–24
Klein M: On identification (1955), in Envy and Gratitude and Other Works, 1946–1963. New York, Delacorte/Seymour Laurence, 1975, pp 141–175
McGuire W (ed): The Freud/Jung Letters: The Correspondence Between Sigmund Freud and C. G. Jung. Princeton, NJ, Princeton University Press, 1974
McLaughlin JT: Clinical and theoretical aspects of enactment. J Am Psychoanal Assoc 39:595–614, 1991
Mitchell SA: Relational Concepts in Psychoanalysis: An Integration. Cambridge, MA, Harvard University Press, 1988
Mitchell SA: Hope and Dread in Psychoanalysis. New York, Basic Books, 1993
Money-Kyrle RE: Normal counter-transference and some of its deviations. Int J Psychoanal 37:360–366, 1956
Ogden TH: On projective identification. Int J Psychoanal 60:357–373, 1979
Ogden TH: Projective Identification and Psychotherapeutic Technique. New York, Jason Aronson, 1982
Ogden TH: The Matrix of the Mind: Object Relations and the Psychoanalytic Dialogue. Northvale, NJ, Jason Aronson, 1986
Ogden TH: The dialectically constituted/decentred subject of psychoanalysis, II: the contributions of Klein and Winnicott. Int J Psychoanal 73:613–626, 1992
Ogden TH: Subjects of Analysis. Northvale, NJ, Jason Aronson, 1994
Racker H: Transference and Countertransference. New York, International Universities Press, 1968
Renik O: Analytic interaction: conceptualizing technique in light of the analyst's irreducible subjectivity. Psychoanal Q 72:553–571, 1993
Renik O: The role of an analyst's expectations in clinical technique: reflections on the concept of resistance. J Am Psychoanal Assoc 43:83–94, 1995
Rosenfeld HA: Notes on the psycho-analysis of the superego conflict of an acute schizophrenic patient. Int J Psychoanal 31:111–131, 1952
Roughton RE: Useful aspects of acting out: repetition, enactment, and actualization. J Am Psychoanal Assoc 41:443–472, 1993
Sandler J: Countertransference and role-responsiveness. International Review of Psychoanalysis 3:43–47, 1976
Sandler J: On communication from patient to analyst: not everything is projective identification. Int J Psychoanal 74:1097–1107, 1993
Segal H: An Introduction to the Work of Melanie Klein. New York, Basic Books, 1964

Spillius EB: Clinical experiences of projective identification, in Clinical Lectures on Klein and Bion. Edited by Anderson R. London, Tavistock/Routledge, 1992, pp 59–73

Tansey MJ: Sexual attraction and phobic dread in the countertransference. Psychoanalytic Dialogue 4:139–152, 1994

Winnicott DW: Hate in the countertransference. Int J Psychoanal 30:69–75, 1949

Chapter 2

Countertransference in the Treatment of the Suicidal Borderline Patient

John T. Maltsberger, M.D.

The many difficulties that borderline patients suffer stem from their central pathology: the incapacity to maintain reasonably stable, separate self and object representations. They tend to mix up fragments of their self representations with those of their objects, getting confused about which traits are theirs and which belong to others. The want of a stable self representation, colored with sufficient positive emotional color to make it narcissistically stable, repeatedly causes them to "go to pieces" and accounts for the dread of abandonment that drives much of their desperate behavior (Stolorow 1975). Their proclivity for defensive splitting, as well as their vulnerability to suicide, rises from instability of the representational self (Maltsberger 1993). This instability makes it impossible to maintain consistently a sense of self and object separateness, and it drives the intense transference and countertransference phenomena that make these patients' psychotherapy so taxing and painful to both patient and therapist.

Borderline patients "go to pieces" both in the everyday and in the technical senses. Behind their brisk mood shifts and dizzying changes of attitude toward others lie friable inner images of themselves and other people. What such a patient acknowledges to be part of himself today he will ascribe to another person tomorrow. Bits of the self-image are broken off and projected into others according to the needs of the moment. Since distortion, projection, and denial are major devices in the defense repertory of borderline patients, it follows that their capacity for reality testing is uncertain and variable. Borderline patients project bits of themselves into others when anxiety rises; as a general rule, the fragmented self-aspects they cast into others are those that if acknowledged as their own would stir up intolerable psychic pain. Dispatching these disturbing parts into others frees the borderline patient of psychic thorns. For instance, if the patient cannot stand to acknowledge he hates someone because the resulting guilt would be intolerable, he jettisons his hating-self, as it were, casting it into the imago of someone else. "It is not that I want to reject you," the formula runs. "You want to reject me." The patient then has the subjective experience of being hated by someone else, though the other person is not, in fact, doing the hating.

How does such a pattern develop? We look first to Melanie Klein's theory. Mrs. Klein believed that in the earliest weeks of life infants separate their experiences of pleasure-contentment and pain-danger into separate compartments of good and bad. The infant retains the "good" as the nucleus of his earliest self representation, whereas the "bad" he tends to disavow (expel) to the outside. As the capacity for self-object differentiation progresses, the maturing child develops a representational system of good me/bad me and good mother/bad mother, the boundaries between which are fluid. Only as reality testing and object constancy are established are the self and object representations more or less stabilized and brought into accord with "reality" (Klein 1946). As the child enters latency he begins to maintain more or less stable self and object representations in which both the good and the bad are integrated, though throughout life even healthy people tend to ward off unpleasant self-aspects by attributing them to others, albeit briefly.

Mahler (1968) developed these ideas, which were taken up in turn by others. Kernberg (1967, 1975) identified splitting as the paramount defense of borderline patients. Splitting operates to keep opposing introjects and the affects attached to them apart, he argued. Splitting is an archaic defensive pattern arising from the time before good and bad part objects are integrated into whole representations that can sustain both positive and negative affects (ambivalence). One of the consequences of the predisposition to splitting is the tendency to divide all objects into two camps—the all-goods and the all-bads. (For a very helpful review of this matter, the reader may wish to turn to the book by Gabbard and Wilkinson [1994], pp. 173–197; see also Chapter 1, this volume.)

The unstable self and object representational system so typical of these patients may well account for their vulnerability to painful states of unreality and depersonalization. They often cannot tell whether they are real or not and often experience their bodies as detached from their very fluid subjective sense of self. They often cut or burn themselves in order to escape these painful affects, concentrating their wounds on the skin. It appears that pain arising from the skin serves to emphasize the physical boundary between self and the outside and helps the patients to "pull themselves together."

Suicidal Borderline Patients

Though the countertransference difficulties borderline patients impose on psychotherapists are formidable, those imposed by patients who threaten or attempt suicide are particularly troublesome. Most borderline patients raise the suicide specter at some point in their treatment, though comparatively few ever go forward to kill themselves. Stone (1990) reported that the suicide rate among patients with borderline personality disorder was 8.9%, whereas McGlashan (1986) estimated this rate to be 3%. Though such patients threaten suicide, injure themselves frequently without actually intending to die, and truly attempt suicide from time to time, most personality disorder patients who commit suicide also suffer from major depression, alcoholism, or drug abuse (Robins et al. 1959). Most borderline patients who kill themselves have comorbid major depression; a clinical impression awaiting empirical validation strongly suggests that those borderline patients with comorbid depression who are at greatest risk experience intense mental anguish (psychic anxiety), powerful self-hate, and a conviction they will never get better (Fawcett 1997; Maltsberger 1997).

Though borderline patients stir up powerful countertransference reactions in those who treat them, suicidal borderline patients give rise to reactions of even more than ordinary difficulty.

The subjective experience of a psychotherapist who suffers through a treatment that does not go well, or even fails, is a different matter from that of the clinician whose patient dies. The anticipation of a patient's possible death is fearful. If the patient dies because of errors in the treatment, the bereaved therapist will have to endure not only grief but also shame. This is precisely what the suicidal borderline patient threatens: "If I am driven to suicide, it will be because of your insufficiency," the patient seems to say. The insufficiencies the patient adduces are various, but all of them are unpleasant—therapists are accused of not caring, of hatefulness, of surrendering hope, of insensitivity, and sometimes of secretly wanting the patient to die.

If a patient dies while blaming the therapist, it is extremely difficult for the therapist not to credit the patient's reproaches, at least at some level, for therapists often join patients in an unconscious way, coming to feel that their treatment maneuvers ought to be omnipotent, even though they know this is impossible. Birtchnell (1983), warning against the danger of the therapist's taking too much responsibility for keeping the patient alive, speculated that excessive anxiety about a patient's possible suicide sometimes reflects a reaction formation against the therapist's own latent suicidal wishes. Birtchnell warns against too great a missionary zeal to "convert" suicidal patients to the therapist's way of thinking.

Whether or not one agrees with Birtchnell, general clinical experience suggests that the threat of losing a patient to suicide arouses abandonment anxiety in the therapist—the same kind of anxiety that torments borderline patients (Gunderson 1984). It may well be that this shared common anxiety invites unconscious identification with the patient, helping projective identification to occur.

Buie (1982) presupposed that the central motivation for most psychotherapists was to derive a secure holding environment in treating patients. He pointed out that the most fundamental need of human beings is the allaying of separation anxiety. As parents may use their children to stabilize a sense of security, so may therapists use patients. Abandonment anxiety would appear not only to derive from preoedipal separation dread but also to be colored by castration anxiety. In mythology, we may recall, the infant Oedipus was left wounded and alone on the side of a mountain to die. He survived to adulthood, but after he discovered that he had unwittingly committed parricide and incest, he wounded himself again (by blinding) and wandered alone and friendless until he died. Inevitably, the dreaded experience of abandonment is associated with a sense of having been bad and is felt to be a punishment. Therapists fearing the loss of a patient to suicide very generally fear that in losing the patient they will be guilty of killing him, or at least of carelessly permitting a needless death.

Omnipotent self-expectations underlie such attitudes, of course, but therapists' fears of banishment, punishment, professional rejection, and malpractice actions are not altogether unrealistic. In many training programs and hospital communities, even though everyone knows that suicide is not always preventable, there is a tendency to feel that such is not so (Maltsberger 1994). Many hospitals now operate under clinical risk management laws requiring systematic investigation of all suicides. Many of these investigations are conducted in an atmosphere where there is a clear presumption that something went wrong or the patient would still be alive. Such proceedings tend to heighten self-blame and omnipotent self-expectation in the suicidally bereaved clinician caught up in them.

Psychological Circumstances Favoring Projective Identification

Projective identification, an interactive phenomenon highly characteristic of all the borderline patient's relationships, lies at the heart of transference-countertransference difficulties in the patient's psychotherapy. Ogden (1979) divided this phenomenon into three phases:

1. The patient wishes to get rid of some self-aspect (including internal objects, or introjects) that threatens to destroy the self from within or that itself seems threatened with destruction and for that reason must be assigned to another person for safekeeping.

2. The patient, projecting the self-aspect into someone else, exerts an influence on the other person to experience himself and to behave in a way congruent with the unconsciously projected material.
3. The person into whom the patient's projections have been directed experiences himself in part as he is pictured in the patient's projective fantasy. In short, the patient throws some aspect of himself into the outside world (projection) and unconsciously contrives that the target at whom he aims introjects it and experiences it to some degree as his own.

I have already suggested that part of the matrix that favors projective identification is the common vulnerability of both patient and therapist to abandonment anxiety. The therapist's abandonment anxiety is likely to crescendo as suicide seems imminent, permanent separation is threatened, and identification with the patient intensifies.

A further phenomenon inviting projective identification is the instability of the self organization of borderline patients and the difficulty they experience in keeping self and object representations separate. McGlashan (1983) showed how this difficulty shapes these patients' transferences: because they tend to fuse self and object representations, their selves are likely to be experienced as the therapeutic relationship. McGlashan refers to this fused representational state as the "we-self" and points out that borderline patients need another person to feel real, whole, or complete, to maintain any sense of continuing temporal identity, to have a sense of having a mind, to have any awareness of feelings, and to have any sense of value or role.

Empathic connection with any patient requires temporary identification with the patient's self-experience, or "trial identification." When working with the borderline patient, the therapist is required to take inside, albeit on a temporary basis, the we-self experience. When both patient and therapist experience abandonment anxiety, it may become difficult for the therapist to let go of the identification that began as an empathic trial. Both patient and therapist can become confused as to who is feeling what, and coercive transference-countertransference bondage results.

Coercive Bondage

Hendin (1981) described a deadly countertransference problem in which the patient succeeds in making the therapist feel more responsible for his survival than the patient does himself. A pattern evolves in which suicide threats and then attempts, often of increasing danger, occur, and in response the therapist rushes into rescue actions. Such behavior by the therapist is characteristically driven by overidentification with the patient, a high level of abandonment anxiety, and reaction formation against the anger aroused by the patient.

Though empathy with the patient's inner experience is essential, the therapist must maintain enough psychic distance to "think his own thoughts"—that is, to have a sufficiently stable self organization so that he does not take over the patient's expectation that he will take full responsibility for the psychic and physical survival of the we-self relationship (Gabbard and Wilkinson 1994). Suicidal patients cannot get better until they accept most of the responsibility for their own living or dying. The therapist who is unprepared to take reasonable risks in order to give the patient appropriate responsibility for self-survival will soon find himself in the type of bondage described by Hendin (1981). The patient must learn that suicidal maneuvers aim to coerce rescue from pain—that is, they are demands for succor as much as they are efforts at dying (Maltsberger 1994). A new language (i.e., spoken words), whereby the patient describes his desperation instead of portraying it through suicidal action, must be learned.

Countertransference Inflation: Reactions to Idealizing Projections

Part of Ogden's (1979) formula for projective identification refers to sending valuable parts of the patient's self into others for safekeeping, lest they be destroyed by other parts of the patient's self. We meet this clinically when the patient "splits" his object representation and conveys both to himself and to the therapist that the therapist is perfect. Such idealization is likely to take place early in treatment; it indicates what the patient wishes the therapist may be. The idealizing attributions typically include perfect empathy ("Nobody has ever understood me so perfectly as you" or "Sometimes you seem to be able to read my mind," the patient may say), extraordinary healing powers ("All the other patients say you are so helpful; you are so much better at this work than my last therapist"), physical attractiveness ("You are so handsome" or "You are so beautiful"), wisdom, and various other agreeable qualities. It is a rare therapist who can hear such blandishments without experiencing some degree of self-inflation, even if he knows what the patient says is not realistic. To the extent that the patient's idealization is introjected, it tends, in Kohut's (1971) language, to inflate the therapist's grandiose self. More classically, we might formulate as follows: That introjection of the patient's idealization interferes with the therapist's reality testing to the extent that he experiences his self representation as coming much closer to his ego-ideal than can truly be the case. The result is a sense of more or less grandiose self-inflation.

The more the therapist truly aspires to be magically empathic, therapeutically omnipotent, and extraordinarily attractive physically, the more impossible will his ego-ideal prove, and the more vulnerable will he be to narcissistic destabilization. We may aspire to be Superman or Wonder Woman in our latency years, but latency remnants in the ego-ideal of psychotherapists always make trouble.

When therapists are vulnerable to grandiose inflation, their reality testing may fail and the stage is set for erotic or other kinds of harmful boundary violations. In such emotional states, therapists feel they are so exceptional that the usual rules that guide their work do not apply.

Countertransference Shock: Reactions to Debasing (Hostile) Projections

Inevitably, with borderline patients, something transpires in the treatment to disappoint the patient, and the debasing side of the split asserts itself. The therapist, perhaps lulled by previous idealizing blandishments, suddenly finds himself accused of profound empathic obtuseness, coldness, indifference, stupidity, personal grotesquerie, or ugliness. The therapeutic honeymoon is suddenly over, and the abrupt turn of events can seem startlingly unfair. Some degree of narcissistic rage (Kohut 1972) will be aroused; if the treatment is not to founder, this rage must be managed with graceful balance.

In speaking of projective identification's second phase, Ogden (1979) commented that the phenomenon does not exist when there is no interaction between projector and recipient. Projective identification does not take place through mystical, unseen transpiration between patient and therapist. Patients do something to their therapists that evokes reactions that validate what they project. Patients may resort to all manner of provocative behaviors (e.g., jostling, keeping prolonged silence, withholding fees, coming late), but a very common, if not universal, device is to insist that the therapist secretly feels or thinks something the therapist does not like and then to evoke precisely that in him. In enticing the therapist to feel especially fine when idealization is projected, the patient plays on the relationship between the therapist's self-perception and his ego-ideal. So it is when debasement is projected. The patient causes the therapist to feel, and even to behave, in ways that evoke countertransference guilt and shame. The therapist introjects the debasement, identifies with it, and may even act it out. He experiences a fall in self-esteem.

The debasing projections the patient unconsciously seeks to intrude into the therapist are organized around the two primary aspects of hate: aversion and malice (Maltsberger and Buie 1973). The patient cannot stand his own wishes to abandon the therapist and tries to get the therapist to do the abandoning. Neither can the patient bear his own sadism; he tries to evoke the therapist's cruelty.

When the therapist acts out his sadistic (malicious) identification with the patient (he may say sarcastic or other stinging things, offer tactlessly blunt interpretations, or otherwise betray impatience), the therapeutic damage will generally be less than when aversion-abandonment projective identifications are acted out. After all, most borderline patients are quite accustomed to sadomasochistic exchanges and appear to tolerate them very well. Their intolerance of abandonment, however, being central to their pathology, is a serious matter. Losing the relationship, especially if a we-self transference has been established, is tantamount to losing one's self (McGlashan 1983).

If borderline patients are better able to tolerate sadistic reactions from their therapists than aversive ones, by and large therapists tolerate patients' aversive feelings better than their sadistic ones. Many physicians (and other psychotherapists) rely heavily on reaction formation against their own sadism and grow very anxious when their malicious potential is aroused. Trainees (and sometimes more experienced therapists) may feel such great distress when unconsciously sadistically excited that they may attempt to distance themselves from patients, even to the extent of interrupting the treatment.

The following example shows how projective identification can stir up aversive acting out in psychotherapists.

> A borderline patient was assigned to a psychiatric resident who was unusually sensitive and repelled by wrist cutting. Tired and overworked, the resident decided to "set limits" when her patient superficially lacerated her own forearm. She told the patient that no more wrist cutting would be tolerated and that if she persisted in it the treatment would have to end. The patient cut herself again a few hours after the session ended and reported this at the next appointment. The therapist thereupon terminated the treatment, and the patient committed suicide.

When this case was reviewed in a postmortem conference, it became painfully clear that the resident had felt very angry at the patient's cutting behavior and could not stand what the patient aroused in her: certainly she felt very helpless. Further, it seemed probable that under her helplessness the resident could not stand the cruel impulses that the patient was generating in her through projective identification. In an effort to reclaim her own equilibrium, this therapist warned the patient that if the cutting did not stop she would interrupt the treatment. This the patient understood to represent a threat of abandonment. She experienced a crescendo of very painful, dissociated suffering and cut herself again in order to relieve the suffering. When, in fact, the treatment abruptly ended, the patient felt abandoned and fell into an intolerable affective state that drove her to suicide.

Not all countertransference is driven by projective identification. Though the following case example does not illustrate projective identification, it does show how a narcissistically wounded therapist can feel destructive and wish to take flight.

> A first-year psychiatry resident, assigned a psychotically depressed, suicidal man, was horrified when the attending psychiatrist suggested the patient receive a course of electroconvulsive treatment. The resident, required to be present when the first seizure was induced, left the room as soon as he could, greatly distressed. Later that day in his own psychoanalytic hour he denounced electroconvulsive treatment as a barbarity, although it was plain that withholding it from this particular patient would probably have resulted in a suicide attempt. He told his analyst he wanted to resign from the case if more electroconvulsive treatment were insisted on by the attending psychiatrist.
>
> Presently the resident noticed that he was not only indignant but also ashamed and quite guilty about having participated in the first treatment. In passing, he mentioned the patient's name. The analyst then asked whether the patient did not have the same first name as the resident's younger brother.
>
> The resident quickly began to recall how he had hated his little brother; he described the constant fighting and minor cruelties that had marred their childhood relationship. He remembered having once choked his brother blue in the face; this he connected to the patient's seizure, and he began to appreciate how much his wish to get off the case was in the service of avoiding reexperiencing his boyhood sadism.

This clinical example shows how the combination of reaction formation and rationalization can permit aversive acting out in the service of keeping malicious fantasies out of mind. The patient had aroused this resident's narcissistic rage, not through the usual direct verbal attacks on his ego-ideal, but through action: The resident's narcissism had been bruised because an omnipotent self-expectation, to get the patient better through developing a therapeutic relationship and prescribing psychoactive drugs, had been thwarted. The patient made him feel helpless, and this made him unconsciously very angry (Sharaf and Levinson 1964).

Psychotherapists who cannot allow sadistic arousal to enter consciousness are apt to decide not to continue treatment with their borderline patients. Sometimes distortion of clinical understanding takes place so that an incorrect decision is made that the patient cannot benefit from psychotherapy and discharge is rationalized. Sometimes patients are transferred to other hospitals because of countertransference aversion.

Counterprojection is another device enabling therapists to disavow unwelcome feelings. Having introjected some of the patient's cruel self through projective identification, and having experienced the harmonic reverberation of his own sadistic potential as a result, the therapist may reproject the intolerable part back into the patient, along with the excitement he has added to it. In these circumstances, therapists sometimes wrongly decide that patients are suicidal according to the formula "I do not want to kill (attack) my patient; the patient wants to kill himself." Hospitalization or other disruption, including transfer of the patient to other caregivers, is common when this occurs.

Empirical investigation of suicides among patients with borderline personality disorder has shown that in a very high proportion of cases, caregivers' rejection behavior preceded the suicide (Kullgren 1988; Kullgren et al. 1986).

The defenses that therapists may call into play to keep their sadism out of mind, all of which invite abandonment of the patient to a greater or lesser degree, are various and have been described elsewhere (Maltsberger and Buie 1973). The kind of interplay described, however, in which ownership of repudiated self-parts can be disavowed by both patient and therapist, threatens psychotherapeutic treatment of borderline patients generally but is particularly dangerous when suicide vulnerability is high.

Enlistment of the Therapist in Suicide

Most clinicians are aware that many patients who commit suicide give direct or indirect indications of what they intend beforehand. Less appreciated is the fact that presuicidal communications are often intended to recruit the permission of others to go ahead with self-killing, or even to evoke the wish in others that the patient might go ahead and finish it. Sometimes family members who have rescued a patient from overdosing too often give up at last and let the patient die from a final ingestion (Richman and Rosenbaum 1970; Wolk-Wasserman 1986). Reports appear from time to time in which someone determined to die provokes his own murder, the equivalent of suicide (Jenet and Segal 1985).

Efforts to recruit others to participate in suicide appear in the interactions between patients and therapists as well (Maltsberger and Buie 1994). Asch (1980) described a suicide complex in which a patient's deadly self-part (he called it "the hidden executioner") is projected into the analyst so that the patient perceives the analyst as wishing him dead. Under such circumstances, the patient unconsciously wishes to punish the therapist, to be punished for his evil wish, and to be cast aside to die. The craving for punishment may become especially intense when the patient grasps that his transference hatred is largely unjustified by adult reality.

A sense of personal security and value requires the laying down of a stable organization of positive introjects through the course of development that must outweigh the dynamic force of whatever destructive ones may also be internalized. Suicide-prone patients have no such system, and therefore they cannot regulate anxiety and maintain stable self-regard without recruiting sustaining external resources, normally other people. Kohut (1971) called such resources "selfobjects."

To the extent that suicide-vulnerable patients can make use of whatever positive introjective resources they have, helped along by benign and dependable exterior sustaining others, they manage to limp along through life, however precariously and anxiously (the threat of abandonment never entirely goes away). When sustaining others withdraw, or seem to do so, the patient's narcissistic integrity is threatened by a rising tide of fear and rage. Projection and distortion make others seem hostile. When others are experienced all of a piece with the abandoning, hating, and devaluating primary objects as represented by intolerable negative introjects, the patient may be driven to suicide to end his suffering, punish the world, and punish himself (Maltsberger 1986).

Unconsciously, determinedly suicidal patients crave validation for their hateful view of others as cruel and abandoning. They expectably will attempt to provoke the therapist to do or say something so that they can rightfully feel wronged. If this validation can be obtained, a suicide attempt can be justified.

> A 27-year-old medical secretary with borderline personality disorder had been in psychotherapy for many years. There had been 14 hospital admissions, repeated body slashings, and 6 dangerous overdoses. Central to her pathology was a malignant bondage to her mother, who appeared in the treatment as a murderous, transference-dominating introject.
>
> Disappointed by not receiving a hoped-for promotion at work, the patient announced to her therapist that she had made a "discovery," namely, that he had never truly cared about her, that he only wanted her money, and that he was a phony trickster and liar. Fortunately the therapist was the master of the ensuing countertransference rage and behaved appropriately. The alliance seemed intact, so he remained quietly attentive, saying nothing, waiting for the patient's storm to subside. Nevertheless, he was aware of a private thought that he wished he was far from her. She lunged and stormed provocatively, then paused and glared at her therapist. She said, "If you yell at me, you'll never see me again!" and then, after a pause, "I think you want me to kill myself."
>
> In the next session, she told her therapist that she had been so enraged at him she wanted to kill herself but that she could not do it alone. The therapist replied, "You want me to help you do it." To this she assented and she quieted down and was able to describe how she wanted violence between herself and the doctor. She wanted him guilty. A few days later she was nearly run over by a car, and, glancing up at the driver as she jumped out of the way, she imagined seeing her therapist as the driver. (Maltsberger and Buie 1994)

Conclusion

The unstable, poorly integrated self representation in the mental structure of patients with borderline personality disorder, with a tendency to confuse parts of the self with object representations, underlies their use of splitting as a defense. It also is responsible for the "we-self" transference (McGlashan 1983) and underlies the phenomenon of projective identification. Therapists frequently share some proclivity for abandonment anxiety with their borderline patients. When suicide is threatened, the therapist's dread of being sent away (the patient may die) becomes a basis for identification with the patient. At such times, empathic trial identification with the patient can lead the therapist into some degree of boundary confusion that leads to coercive bondage.

Patients tend to give therapists most (or all) of the responsibility for keeping them alive when this happens, and unless the bondage relationship is resolved, suicide is likely. Suicidal patients need to take most of the responsibility for their own living if they are to make headway in psychotherapy.

Projective identification is possible because of the patient's influence on the therapist's narcissism. When idealizing projections are taken in, the therapist is in danger of grandiose inflation—of supposing the usual constraints and boundaries of psychotherapy can be set aside. This leads to the danger of erotic and other intimate acting out. When the patient assaults the therapist's narcissism with debasing projections, the therapist must experience some degree of narcissistic rage. If he cannot tolerate the conscious experience of his own sadism, he is at risk of acting out aversively, abandoning the patient, and precipitating a suicide.

Patients also may project a lethal introject into therapists, attempting to enlist the therapist as an ally, or an accomplice, in the suicidal act. Acute sensitivity to this process and care not to validate such projections are essential in preventing patient suicide.

References

Asch SS: Suicide and the hidden executioner. International Review of Psycho-Analysis 7:51–60, 1980

Birtchnell J: Psychotherapeutic considerations in the management of the suicidal patient. Am J Psychother 37:24–36, 1983

Buie DH: The abandoned therapist. International Journal of Psychoanalytic Psychotherapy 9:227–232, 1982

Fawcett J: The detection and consequences of anxiety in clinical depression. J Clin Psychiatry 58 (no 8, suppl):35–40, 1997

Gabbard GO, Wilkinson SM: Management of Countertransference With Borderline Patients. Washington, DC, American Psychiatric Press, 1994

Gunderson JG: Borderline Personality Disorder. Washington, DC, American Psychiatric Press, 1984

Hendin H: Psychotherapy and suicide. Am J Psychother 35:469–480, 1981

Jenet RN, Segal RJ: Provoked shooting by police as a mechanism for suicide. Am J Forensic Med Pathol 6:274–275, 1985

Kernberg O: Borderline personality organization. J Am Psychoanal Assoc 15:641–685, 1967

Kernberg OF: Borderline Conditions and Pathological Narcissism. New York, Jason Aronson, 1975

Klein M: Notes on some schizoid mechanisms (1946), in Envy and Gratitude and Other Works, 1946–1963. New York, Delacorte/Seymour Laurence, 1975, pp 1–24

Kohut H: The Analysis of the Self: A Systematic Approach to the Psychoanalytic Treatment of Narcissistic Personality Disorders. New York, International Universities Press, 1971

Kohut H: Thoughts on narcissism and narcissistic rage. Psychoanal Study Child 27:360–402, 1972

Kullgren G: Factors associated with completed suicide in borderline personality disorder. J Nerv Ment Dis 176:40–44, 1988

Kullgren G, Renberg E, Jacobsson L: An empirical study of borderline personality disorder and psychiatric suicides. J Nerv Ment Dis 174:328–331, 1986

Mahler MS: On Human Symbiosis and the Vicissitudes of Individuation, Vol 1: Infantile Psychosis. New York, International Universities Press, 1968

Maltsberger JT: Suicide Risk: The Formulation of Clinical Judgment. New York, New York University Press, 1986

Maltsberger JT: Confusions of the body, the self, and others in suicidal states, in Suicidology: Essays in Honor of Edwin Shneidman. Edited by Leenaars A. Northvale, NJ, Jason Aronson, 1993, pp 148–171

Maltsberger JT: Calculated risks in the treatment of intractably suicidal patients. Psychiatry 57:199–212, 1994

Maltsberger JT: Ecstatic suicide. Archives of Suicide Research 3: 283–301, 1997

Maltsberger JT, Buie DH: Countertransference hate in the treatment of suicidal patients. Arch Gen Psychiatry 30:625–633, 1973

Maltsberger JT, Buie DH: The psychotherapist as an accomplice in suicide. Italian Journal of Suicidology 4:75–81, 1994
McGlashan TH: The "we-self" in borderline patients: manifestations of the symbiotic self-object in psychotherapy. Psychiatry 46:351–361, 1983
McGlashan TH: The Chestnut Lodge Follow-Up Study, III: long-term outcome of borderline personalities. Arch Gen Psychiatry 43:20–30, 1986
Ogden TH: On projective identification. Int J Psychoanal 60:357–373, 1979
Richman J, Rosenbaum M: A clinical study of the role of hostility and death wishes by the family and society in suicidal attempts. Israel Annals of Psychiatry and Related Disciplines 8:213–231, 1970
Robins E, Murphy GE, Wilkinson RH, et al: Some clinical considerations in the prevention of suicide based on a study of 134 successful suicides. Am J Public Health 49:888–889, 1959
Sharaf MR, Levinson DJ: The quest for omnipotence in professional training: the case of the psychiatric resident. Psychiatry 27:135–149, 1964
Stolorow RD: Toward a functional definition of narcissism. Int J Psychoanal 56:179–185, 1975
Stone MH: The Fate of Borderline Patients. New York, Guilford, 1990
Wolk-Wasserman D: Suicidal communication of persons attempting suicide and responses of significant others. Acta Psychiatr Scand 73: 481–499, 1986

Chapter 3

Countertransference in General Psychiatry

Marcia Kraft Goin, M.D.

> *The working distresses of psychiatrists are rarely fully conscious or owned openly, and almost never discussed as facts which merit scientific study. Rather they are suppressed, even repressed as something we must rise above, something professionally shameful. (Main 1977, p. 462)*

Since 1910, when Freud (1910/1957) first concerned himself with therapists' emotional responses to their patients, many papers on the subject of countertransference have been published. *Countertransference*—defined in *Psychoanalytic Terms and Concepts* as a phenomenon referring "to the attitudes and feelings, only partly conscious, of the analyst towards the patient" (Moore and Fine 1968, p. 29)—plays a major role in shaping psychiatrists' reactions in many aspects of their work. Although technically understood to be a natural presence and process in the treatment setting, countertransference is experienced by many clinicians as an uncomfortable "foreign object." A reflection of this discomfort surfaced during a study observing 24 psychoanalysts supervising psychiatric residents (Goin and Kline 1976). The researchers, after analyzing videotapes of these sessions, were surprised to find that the supervisors avoided discussion of even the most obvious countertransference issues. This avoidance persisted even when the residents raised questions and concerns about the subject. Perhaps this is not so surprising. Although it is known that countertransference enhances our awareness of patients' pathology and provides clues to diagnosis and patients' conflicts, countertransference still points a finger at therapists' emotions that are contrary to the idealized image of the ever-empathic and understanding physician.

Over the years, countertransference has been characterized in a number of ways (Tyson 1986). At one end of the spectrum, countertransference is said to mean only the therapist's transference reactions to the patient's transference. At the other extreme, it refers to all of a caretaker's affects, thoughts, fantasies, and behaviors, conscious and unconscious, that occur with patients. In this chapter I use the following broad definition: all of the therapist's feelings and reactions to patients, including troublesome feelings that can sabotage treatment and make the therapist miserable, and other feelings that provide useful clues to understanding the patient's mental processes and conflicts. These feelings may be raw, intense, and very much within the clinician's conscious perception. They may also be subtle or masked expressions of affects that are outside the psychiatrist's conscious awareness.

A survey by Plutnick and colleagues (1994) suggests that more experienced therapists are less defensive and more open to appreciating both the helpful and the disruptive manifestations of countertransference. In their work, these authors looked at what they called "critical incidents in psychiatry": situations that an unbiased observer would expect to provoke some type of emotional response. Experienced psychiatrists and psychiatric residents were asked to report on the frequency of such occurrences as well as their interpretations of the importance for five categories of interaction or behavior. The five categories were threat of harm from the patient, criticism of the therapist or the therapy, occurrence of a major life crisis, attempts by the patient to seek friendship or seduction, and miscellaneous incidents such as being consistently late. Plutnick et al. were looking to see if there was a difference between experienced psychiatrists and psychiatric residents in terms of recognition and appreciation of these items. They found that although the residents identified patients as exhibiting these behaviors more frequently than did experienced psychiatrists, the residents did not identify such issues as being particularly important. It is hoped that the information in this chapter will provide a useful distillation of clinical wisdom.

Countertransference reactions are an expected natural occurrence in our work with patients. Some of these are the automatic human responses provoked by hostile, dangerous, or tragic events; others are reactions to the patient's psychopathology or character style; and still others are products of our own personal history. These reactions can occur almost anywhere—in the privacy of a consultation room, in the psychiatric hospital or emergency room, while walking down the corridor of a medical ward, or while consulting in the jail. We may be aware of these feelings, or we may become aware of them only when situations such as forgetting appointments or neglecting to renew a prescription signal their presence. Wherever they occur and whatever their psychological origin, accepting their presence helps to make us their master and enhances the therapeutic process.

Medication Compliance

As effective as a medication may be, it is worthless if the patient does not take it. However skilled and knowledgeable a psychiatrist may be about medications, including side effects and drug-drug interactions, the knowledge has little therapeutic value if the patient fails to comply with the physician's recommendation.

Patients' noncompliance with medications and other prescribed treatment programs has long been recognized as a major obstacle to the physician's ability to provide good health care. A recent review of the literature by Cramer and Rosenheck (1998) confirmed the existence of this problem and the observation that psychiatric patients have even greater problems with compliance than do patients with medical disorders. Examining the research on compliance, they found that the mean compliance rate for patients with physical disorders was 76%, with a range from 60% to 92%. Psychiatric patients, on the other hand, had an average of 58% compliance, with a range from 24% to 92%.

In dealing with this problem, we are helped by our knowledge of human behavior but often especially challenged by patients' symptoms and other manifestations of their illness. Symptoms such as paranoia, impulsivity, delusions, and hallucinations can be major impediments to a psychiatrist's efforts in developing a working alliance and compliance with a therapeutic regimen. Similarly, a patient's characterological traits and/or psychodynamic conflicts may interfere with the patient's ability to collaborate with the treatment endeavors and therapeutic recommendations. Dynamic conflicts such as competition with authority, fear of dependence, shaky self-esteem, a sense of entitlement, embarrassment, and defiance represent but a few of such problems. Each of these can pose a problem for the patient when acceptance of the psychiatrist's recommendations is important.

Each of these may also pose a problem for the psychiatrist when the patient's pattern is one that the psychiatrist finds particularly painful, guilt evoking, or noxious. Many examples of such countertransference reactions can be seen when cases of "difficult" and "noncompliant" patients are presented at the outpatient clinical case conference. The following case illustrates this point.

> The case of a 26-year-old unemployed single man living with his mother was presented at the case conference because of his refractoriness to treatment. He had been a patient at the clinic for 18 months, having sought treatment for severe obsessive thoughts and compulsive behaviors. He described being immobilized by the rituals he needed to perform constantly and intense anxiety provoked by his guilty thoughts. Although anxious to be seen by his assigned psychiatric resident, he was consistently late for appointments, but once there he did not want to leave; when he did not believe he was receiving the help he needed, he would demand to be seen by the resident's supervisor. Worried about side effects, he had discontinued each medication that was prescribed before there was an opportunity for the drug to reach a therapeutic level. He refused to attend a group for cognitive therapy because of fear of being contaminated by the group members. Also, he insisted that his obsessive thoughts made it impossible for him to comply with any cognitive or behavioral homework.
>
> As happens in a clinic setting, he was seen over time by a number of different psychiatric residents. The first therapist responded to his irregular attendance and demands for more attention by scheduling frequent appointments each week and constantly readjusting his schedule to try to accommodate the patient's erratic behavior, believing that if he only tried hard enough

he could meet the patient's needs. The next therapist, reviewing the patient's lack of progress and somewhat annoyed by the patient's attitude, tried to insist that the patient follow a rigid schedule of weekly visits. This led to telephone calls to supervisors and the eventual transfer to another therapist, who presented his case at the case conference. At this conference, the therapist commented that he had begun to dread the patient's visits, knowing that he would be left with a terrible sense of failure, responsibility, and guilt over his inability to engage the patient well enough to help relieve the patient's intense psychological pain.

Those in attendance had a variety of reactions to the information about the patient's behavior. It was variously suggested that the patient had "borderline traits," "a sense of entitlement," "severe dependence," and an "antisocial personality disorder." Not surprisingly, the patient, although having agreed to be interviewed at the case conference, telephoned at the last minute to say he was sick and could not leave home.

The patient's problems demonstrate the countertransference reactions that arise in response to patients' resistance to treatment. One could hear in the residents' and staff's responses to the patient's reported behavior expressions of anger, frustration, empathic pain, and guilt. If not recognized and understood, each could lead to nontherapeutic reactions. Some residents would have a tendency to bend in every way imaginable to do the impossible. Others would distance themselves by limiting contact, insisting the patient abide by a contract, demanding an unrealistic level of compliance, and labeling the patient as "borderline" or "too dependent." Still others might be immobilized by their overidentification with the patient's pain.

After the countertransference reactions were aired, a consensus about the problem emerged. Two matters were important to recognize: this patient, although not psychotic, was still very sick, and therapeutic relief was probably going to be quite limited and slow in coming and heavily dependent on the treating psychiatrist's being clinically sensitive to these two facts. The patient's "demanding" and "noncompliant" behavior appeared to be driven by the intense anxieties his symptoms evoked, not by a narcissistic sense of entitlement or ungratified dependent needs to cling. The severity of his illness suggested that successful treatment might be limited or impossible, especially since the options for hospitalization today are so limited. An appropriate plan was outlined that included informing the patient of the limitations of what treatment can offer as well as of the reality of the psychiatrist's time constraints. But it was obvious that the major hurdle in this case would be the challenge of the evoked countertransference reactions.

Psychiatrists need to know themselves and their own personal reactions to the particular behaviors that have the potential to trigger nontherapeutic reactions. Patients who are not psychotic, and therefore appear to be more in control of their behavior, are especially likely to provoke uncomfortable reactions in psychiatrists because their psychological pain is often more disguised and their psychopathology is more obscure. It is easier to appreciate that there is nothing "personal" in the resistance or reluctance to take medication when the patient's reasoning is obstructed by psychotic delusions and disorganization. This is not to say that psychotic patients do not activate countertransference reactions. It is still not uncommon to feel a surge of anger when psychotic patients spit out their medication, hide it, or in some other way sabotage the psychiatrist's recommendations. But as we move up the diagnostic ladder to where there is less ego fragility and disorganization, we are more likely to personalize patients' reactions.

As much as the psychiatrist might know about a patient's history of abuse, desertion, and tragic early life that has led to generalized distrust of everyone, the reality that the patient does not trust his psychiatrist can still be difficult to accept (Goin 1998). Compassionate psychiatrists often need to be reminded that patients will react to them and their prescriptions as they have always reacted to others. If patients are paranoid, they will be paranoid. If they are hypomanic and irresponsible, the same behavior will be seen in their compliance with medical recommendations. If they have obsessive fears about contamination and becoming contaminated, they will live out the same fears in the psychiatrist's office.

Clinicians' unconscious negative or positive feelings can intrude in subtle ways into medication decisions and the timing of return appointments. Patients' psychological as well as medical needs must always be part of the decision when the clinician is titrating the number of pills to be prescribed and determining the frequency of patients' visits—for example, small amounts of medication when frequent visits are deemed mandatory, and larger amounts when there is confidence that the patient is stable and can manage the distance responsibly. Unrecognized and unmonitored countertransference reactions can result in timing that reflects primarily the therapist's wish for distance or a stance that is either unnecessarily or excessively protective. Self-reflection must be an ongoing process, and without this process it is impossible to avoid damaging countertransference blunders.

The considerations addressed here about the psychological responses to pharmacotherapy also apply to electroconvulsive therapy and other somatic therapies.

Split Treatment: The Triangular Relationship

Providing medication consultation and psychopharmacological treatment for patients of a nonmedical psychotherapist is a situation loaded with the potential for "splitting"—on the part of patients and their psychotherapists and psychiatrists. *Splitting* used in this context refers to the psychological mechanism of defense in which there is a polarization of good feelings and bad feelings, of love and hate, and of attachment and rejection. This eventuates in certain people's being seen as all good and others' as all bad. When not recognized, it can lead to polarization of the involved treatment team, hospital staff, or others within the circle who take on these projections and begin to behave as though they are the idealized good person who now must fight on behalf of the patient against the demeaned other.

The configuration of split treatment is increasingly a part of psychiatric practice, and it is therefore imperative to be aware of potential pitfalls. Patients can have any of a number of reactions to this arrangement. They may have negative or positive idealized thoughts and fantasies about medication and the doctors who prescribe it. The physician may be experienced as the authoritarian parent, as the longed-for good parent that never was, as an intruder in a previously private relationship with the psychotherapist, or sometimes as the person he really is. For each reaction there is a potential conscious or unconscious emotional response on the part of each caregiver. Thus, it is necessary to understand and appreciate what Busch and Gould (1993) label the "therapeutic triangle" and the need to achieve what Kahn (1991) describes as a "triadic therapeutic alliance." Split treatment is a natural setting for the replication of the mother-father-child triad, with all of the associated potentials for success or failure. When parenting works well, the parents have a sense of mutual respect for each other. They are open and communicating and both attend to the youngster with care and concern. Problems arise when there is competition, disrespect, and communication failure. The wish to be the favored parent may be acted out, and therapeutically destructive power struggles ensue. It is easy to see how the situation of split treatment, if not carefully monitored, could result in analogous problems.

Beitman and colleagues (1984) point out that most psychiatrists are accustomed to being the primary therapist. The transition to being part of a team, and in particular not the person to whom the patient is principally attached, requires containment of one's usual role and natural narcissism. Although not the primary therapist, the psychiatrist must still work to develop a therapeutic relationship. The importance of this relationship is not diminished by the "triangular" treatment situation. As the relationship develops, an interest in and an attachment to the patient evolve, and reactions are inevitable. The fact that someone else is doing the psychotherapy does not provide immunity to such reactions.

A number of reactions have been highlighted as potential vulnerabilities in this three-way relationship. Busch and Gould (1993) believe that the major countertransference stumbling block is the temptation to collude with the patient's negative transference. Often this occurs in response to two possible sources. The psychopharmacologist may feel narcissistically injured by having to share power with the psychotherapist, harboring a competitive belief that his or her approach is the superior one. The psychiatrist may be made anxious by having to share control of the patient's case. Kahn (1991) notes that in the worst scenario the countertransference struggle may reduce the patient to a narcissistic object while the two therapists struggle for power.

Intergenerational differences can make for additional tensions. When the split treatment involves an older therapist and a younger psychiatrist, or vice versa, both must be particularly alert to the possibility of negative and competitive feelings.

A number of useful strategies have been used to keep these problems from occurring. It is very important to know and respect the referring psychotherapist. This process entails talking together about cases and the psychiatrist's learning how the therapist thinks about clinical issues. If the therapist is unfamiliar with the prescribed medication, it is useful for the psychiatrist to explain about the expected length of time before it takes effect, possible side effects, and drug interactions. The therapist is then familiar with the strengths and the limitations of what is being used and can listen in an educated manner for indications of possible complicating side effects. Communication is essential. Currently, this type of communication is generally not reimbursed by third-party payers. Those who pay for the treatment need to be educated about the importance of this time spent working together and how lack of communication negatively affects the ability to provide high-quality patient care.

The patient needs to be aware that communication between therapist and psychiatrist is taking place. Knowledge of such communication may have an impact on the psychotherapy and needs to be dealt with in that setting. In a situation in which there is mutual respect and communication, the triangular transferences can be anticipated and understood, and the triangular countertransferences can be acknowledged, without embarrassment or damage to the treatment.

Multiple-Treater Settings

The use of the hospital as a curative force has been one of the major casualties in this era of severe cost-containment. In years past, the hospital was a place of safety and security where patients could expose and explore their affects and interactions and make mistakes and learn from them. Today, there is no time for much patient learning to take place. However, the hospital staff and milieu, which can provide a temporary haven and a protective force to which the patient can attach, if ever so fleetingly, continue to have value. Hospitalization is now, by necessity, brief. It does not help that it is the most severely disturbed patients who are now admitted to the hospital and for whom we must find quick solutions. Despite the short length of inpatient treatment, the hospital can still have a therapeutic effect. Pi and colleagues (1983) demonstrated that in as little as 1 week of hospitalization, even acutely symptomatic patients often show significant improvement. In some of these cases, patients experienced a complete remission of symptoms without medication.

The ingredients of the curative force of hospitalization have been conceptualized by Adshead (1998) in terms of attachment theory. In this paradigm, patients experience relief by metaphorically being able to cling temporarily to the safety and security of the hospital and its staff. The hospital cannot serve as a place of security, available for temporary attachment and warmth, if the staff has difficulty tolerating either the external demands of the system or the internal demands of the patient.

The therapeutic relationship between the staff and the patients is described by Gabbard (1992) as central to the healing force of hospitalization. These relationships are often repetitions and re-creations of internal object relations. Therapeutic responses from the clinical staff provide mutative healing ingredients. Splitting and projective identification, in which staff members are experienced as the "bad object," are a frequent occurrence. It is crucial that staff members have continual opportunities to process all of the interactions and reactions that take place.

Certain behaviors signal negative countertransference reactions. On hearing the use of pejorative or dismissive terms to describe a patient, such as "attention seeking," "troublesome," "dependent," or "manipulative," one might suspect that the psychiatric personnel are trying to distance themselves from the discomfort caused by the patient's neediness. When the staff members are overwhelmed by their own unconscious aggressive feelings, this may be covertly masked by the use of professional structures such as rigid enforcement of rules and regulations or inappropriate use of seclusion.

Today's intense focus on cost containment intrudes in myriad ways into our work with patients. Economic forces are increasingly shaping how much time will be made available for treatment, how many days in the hospital will be allowed, how many outpatient visits will be authorized, and what medications can be prescribed. An ever-increasing amount of professional time is spent justifying treatment and obtaining authorization from outside reviewers. Hospital staffs feel pressured to limit the hospital stay and care of very sick patients. It is not difficult to understand how anger with "the system" can at times be displaced onto patients. A ripple effect may occur as frustration with a seemingly irrational authority is turned, consciously or unconsciously, toward the next available target. The patient then reacts to the staff's displaced anger. In the era of managed care, we must be alert to this possibility in order to avoid the damaging ramifications.

Gabbard and colleagues (1991) noted that the opposite can also occur. The staff may collude with the patient in projecting all of the badness onto the insurance reviewer, thereby neglecting important treatment issues. The temptation to do this is particularly strong when the staff is working with patients who are angry and hostile. In the search to achieve some sort of alliance, joining together to attack a common enemy, the insurance company, can seem a ready solution. However, as Gabbard et al. note, such an approach is doomed to fail because the alliance is built on the shaky foundation of splitting and projected hate: "It is only a matter of time until the tables are turned and the treaters are once again regarded as the patient's bad objects" (Gabbard et al. 1991, p. 320). Gabbard et al. speculate that this may be why some patients choose to sue the physician rather than the insurance company.

The organizational structure of the hospital can also be a source of trouble. The interdisciplinary team typically consists of several members, each with different roles and power: staff psychiatrists, residents, nurses, social workers, occupational therapists, and psychologists. Butterill and colleagues (1992) described a number of common problems that develop in this setting. These include confused accountability, poor leadership, a breakdown in communication, and boundary violations such as those felt with the intrusions of managed care. Each of these can initiate or potentiate severe treatment problems. The common thread that these authors described in these examples is that of unconscious displacement of the problem onto the patient. Such displacement can be minimized by the interdisciplinary team's or staff's working together to elucidate and resolve these problems.

A study by Colson and colleagues (1986) collected data about the kinds of reactions patients with particular problems evoked from members of the staff. Among their findings were the following:

1. Patients with a high degree of character pathology (highly demanding, manipulative, hostile, impulsive, sabotaging of treatment) predominately evoked angry reactions. Staff members tended to expect more of these patients than they should have given the patients' ego deficits.
2. Psychotically withdrawn patients produced feelings of helplessness and confusion on the part of the staff as well as a less conspicuous tendency to feel anger and to be provocative. As Main (1957, p. 129) wrote, "The sufferer who frustrates a keen therapist by failing to improve is always in danger of meeting primitive human behavior described as treatment."
3. Suicidal and depressed patients tended to evoke positive interest and protectiveness.
4. Patients who were violent or agitated evoked markedly different affects among the different disciplines. The psychiatrists (all men) felt helpless and confused; the social workers (primarily women) described fearfulness and, paradoxically, a sense of possible engagement; activity therapists felt angry and provoked; and nurses (primarily women) reported being fearful. This variation in reactions among the different disciplines can lead to difficulty for the team in its attempts to develop a cohesive treatment plan for such patients. The greater the awareness of these differences, the greater the likelihood that the team will be able to resolve them in favor of the best treatment plan based on the patient's needs. The authors did not elaborate on the gender differences (men feeling helpless and women feeling fearful). One can speculate that the men's

feelings of helplessness would lead to efforts to take control, a reaction that might be quite appropriate to the situation or unnecessarily rigid. Likewise, the women's fear could lead to suitably protective measures or other maneuvers that are inappropriately distant. Both reactions, when processed in a constructive way, can lead to effective therapeutic measures; if unmonitored, however, these reactions can have destructive effects.

Violent and Assaultive Patients

Psychiatrists are somewhat averse to addressing the subject of psychiatric patients' potential for violence and assaultive behavior directed at their doctors. In part, this aversion arises from concern that focusing on this aspect of behavior will increase the stigma that already accompanies the diagnosis of mental illness. However, this is not the only reason. By minimizing the existence of the problem, the psychiatrist diminishes his or her fears about personal safety. Also, denial of the problem can mask and temporarily soothe discomfort about one's own aggression. All of these factors can contribute to a dangerous avoidance of a hazardous reality.

It is essential to be alert to possible threats, marginal or implicit, and to appreciate one's feelings about patients who are potentially violent or assaultive. Confrontation with assaultive patients stirs fear and even transient feelings of powerlessness in even the most experienced clinicians. To be effective in our treatment efforts, we cannot deny the existence of the problem, nor can we defend ourselves by erecting physical or psychological barriers. Instead, we must protect ourselves primarily with knowledge, keen insight, and self-awareness.

Several studies have addressed the prevalence of violence among psychiatric patients. Swanson and colleagues (1990) conducted a major investigation in which 10,000 inhabitants in three metropolitan communities were interviewed to assess the rate of violent behavior in psychiatric patients. Assaultive behavior was 5 times greater in those with an Axis I diagnosis than in community residents without these diagnoses. Alcohol and/or drug abuse increased the incidence to 10 to 15 times greater than that in the general population. Although most Axis I diagnoses were associated significantly with violent behavior, when those with no comorbid conditions were eliminated from consideration, only schizophrenia (4 times greater than in the general population) and substance abuse (10 times greater) showed a strikingly higher incidence. The MacArthur Violence Risk Assessment Study (Steadman et al. 1998) also demonstrated the effect of substance abuse in increasing the prevalence of violence. In the year after discharge from the hospital, the prevalence of violence among psychiatric patients with coexisting substance abuse and major mental illness was 31.1% compared with 17.9% among those with major mental illness and no substance abuse.

Of considerable clinical interest were findings in a large-scale study by Asnis and colleagues (1997) of 517 patients requesting treatment in an outpatient clinic. The prevalence of self-reported homicide attempts in this population was 4%. Homicidal ideation was more prevalent (22%) than actual homicide attempts. There were no differences between men and women regarding ideation and attempts; the authors speculated that this lack of gender difference was due to the uniform presence of substance abuse. A striking finding was the relationship between homicidal and suicidal ideation: 91% of patients who had attempted homicide also had attempted suicide, and 86% of patients with homicidal ideation also reported suicidal ideation. For those of us who work with patients who have entertained homicidal ideas, this finding comes as no surprise. The authors, in their review, did not find a definite association between specific psychiatric disorders and violent behavior except for substance abuse and antisocial personality, which were associated with an increased risk of violent behaviors.

Swartz and colleagues (1998) examined the effects of substance abuse and noncompliance with prescribed medication and their relationship to violence in the severely mentally ill. They found that the co-occurrence of substance abuse and medication noncompliance made it more than twice as likely that the individual would commit a violent act than when only one of these problems was present.

How active are psychiatrists in evaluating and working to moderate their patients' aggressive behavior? In reviewing material from the session preceding an attack, Dubin and colleagues (1988) found that 39% of the psychiatrists, when looking back on what had occurred in the session prior to being attacked, believed that there was significant information that could have predicted the assault. We must realize, of course, that when reviewing such clinical impressions after the fact, one may overly emphasize the meaning of isolated data. Hindsight is not necessarily missed insight. A very disturbing, but also important, fact is that 21% of the psychiatrists who continued to see the patients after being attacked never discussed the assaultive behavior with the patient (see Chapter 4, this volume).

Dubin (1989) believes that the denial often utilized in these situations is a very dangerous mechanism of defense. He suggests that the staff may avoid inquiring about the patient's homicidal and assaultive thoughts and behaviors for fear that the asking will unleash unmanageable rage. This is similar to a commonly held myth that asking for information about suicidal thoughts increases a patient's risk of suicide. What is important is the manner in which one asks as well as the balanced way in which one responds to the patient's answers. Madden and colleagues (1976) had also found that in the face of threatening information psychiatrists often avoid following up with the specific questions that would help to clarify risk. In their survey of psychiatrists who had been attacked, when the psychiatrists looked back on the sessions prior to tahe assault, 55% of them could see that the patient had reported feelings indicating a potential for violence against the treating psychiatrist. Again, this was material the treaters had failed to follow up on or to clarify.

Lion and colleagues (1976), in their report of a 3-year experience running a violence clinic, highlighted some of the difficulties created for therapists and hospital staffs by mishandling of assaultive and violent behaviors. A number of instructive vignettes are included in this report. In one, the staff, overwhelmed by a patient's assaultive and self-mutilating behavior, had intensified the problem by isolating the patient. Avoidance had seemed preferable to confrontation, but this isolation only served to increase the potential for aggressive behavior. Also, medication had been given only in response to violent outbursts rather than in a consistent and measured manner. As a consequence, the patient had been either violent or insensible. Consultation and open discussion of these matters helped the staff to recognize that alienation from the patient was increasing the psychotic and assaultive potential. They also understood the need to use medications to help the patient modulate her affects and not simply to render her helpless. One would suspect that the clinicians, at some level, knew this before they asked for the consultation—"knew this" in the sense that it was stored somewhere in their warehouse of clinical knowledge. The consultant's advice helped them to neutralize their rage at the patient, and this in turn enabled them to recognize the issues and to respond therapeutically to the patient's behavior. The consultation also gave them a chance to talk about the very real feelings of fear and helplessness that are normal reactions in the face of violence.

Dubin (1989) described a consultation request in response to an "outbreak of violence" in a distant hospital. The consultation revealed a complicated and understaffed clinical situation, with dissension created by staff splitting. Dubin believes that the staff's use of "euphemistic phrases," such as "a problem exists with regard to the acting out of the patients," obscured the true level of violence. It is his contention that this avoidance of a dangerous reality reflected the staff's feelings about violence and their own inability to express violent fantasies and urges. Whatever the etiology, hospital staffs need to recognize when danger is present and if it is escalating. As Dubin reported, patients' angry explosions do not usually come out of the blue; rather, they are in response to subtle insults and unrecognized punitive reactions that develop out of the staff's frustration, anxiety, or unconscious rage. When the prodromal events of an outburst are appropriately identified by both staff and patient, it is possible to handle the feelings differently and to avoid outbursts.

The first task in dealing with potentially assaultive patients is to assess the situation realistically and dispassionately. Any indication that a patient has violent thoughts or is likely to engage in assaultive behavior should be explored in the same careful and thorough manner that one would investigate any other aspect of a patient's mental status. If in the course of an interview a patient volunteers a comment about feeling potentially assaultive, the psychiatrist should ask open-ended as well as specific questions about these feelings and actions. For instance, if a patient says, "I was really angry with my girlfriend last night," an appropriate open-ended question (e.g., "What happened?") should follow. If the described scenario warrants further investigation, it makes sense for the psychiatrist to ask, "Did you feel like hitting her?" or "Did you hit her?" If the patient says yes, then more specific questions to assess the reality are in order. (Examples are "Where did you hit her?" "Was she unconscious?" "Did she have to go to the hospital?" and "Can you see the effects of your hitting her?") These details will not usually be volunteered. Coping with his or her own uneasiness and distaste for such behavior, the psychiatrist will ask questions with careful neutrality. Patients are usually responsive and often relieved by getting the problem out in the open. The fact that the psychiatrist has heard the worst and is still willing to work with them is proof that the therapist is not asking these questions as a moralistic or punitive parent but as a psychiatrist. This approach strengthens the sense of the psychiatrist's reliability. By avoiding a rush to judgment, the psychiatrist encourages the continued development of the therapeutic alliance.

Patients who are psychotic, and particularly those who are paranoid, can be very frightening. Dubin (1989) described a psychiatrist who would not listen or talk to a paranoid schizophrenic patient who telephoned voicing homicidal threats. In reviewing the patient's course, the consultant could see that these threats had escalated during the sessions from bantering to joking threats to, eventually, hostile remarks. None of these threats had been followed up or explored with the patient. The consultant believed that increasing intimacy had resulted in the escalation of the patient's fear and consequent threats. Whatever the dynamic, the psychiatrist needed to recognize and resolve his wish to withdraw. He could then communicate directly and realistically with his patient while meeting with him in a safe environment.

Violence against psychiatrists needs to be reflected on and

talked about freely, openly, and often. In today's world of short hospital stays, closures of psychiatric units in general hospitals, limited outpatient resources, and increasing comorbid illness associated with substance abuse, we have a special mandate to pursue the issue of violence. We tell our patients that talking about fears and feelings of helplessness will not make them worse but instead will give us, the psychiatrists, the means to recognize, analyze, and harness them. The same holds true for feelings about violence.

Consultation and Liaison

The consultation-liaison psychiatrist must contend with a number of issues and perform numerous tasks in addition to the assessment and treatment of patients. Unless the consultant's value is appreciated, the medical or surgical ward is not a friendly place. The physicians in charge have usually exhausted their time-worn nostrums when they finally request a consultation. Frustration with recalcitrant, hostile, or suicidal patients may be displaced onto the consulting psychiatrist, who now must deal therapeutically with both the patient and the medical personnel. Many nonpsychiatric colleagues are uneasy in the world of psychiatry and find it a strange and scary place. Most medical schools do not offer an informative and coherent curriculum about psychiatric diagnosis and treatment, so medical peers often have a limited knowledge of the field. Unfortunately, this combination of stress, incomplete knowledge, and helplessness can lead to hostility and a demeaning attitude toward psychiatry and psychiatrists. Annoyance, rage, hurt, or feelings of humiliation must all be put aside by the psychiatric consultant as the work is redirected toward the task of developing a therapeutic relationship with both staff and patient.

In today's world, hospital staffs are sorely pressed to discharge patients as quickly as possible. Such pressures have always existed, but they are now even more powerful because of the increased focus on cost containment. These forces influence the staff's assessment of the patient. The wish to please, impress, or change our medical colleagues' attitudes can potentially influence our evaluation of the patient and our subsequent recommendations. The consulting psychiatrist must be cautious not to push the patient too fast or too hard, prescribe more psychopharmacological medication than is clearly indicated, or react in other ways that are responses to systemic inequities rather than to the patient's true needs.

The consultation psychiatrist is often needed to assist the whole hospital team in its understanding and treatment of the patient. The patient for whom the consultation is requested may be the "designated patient," but at times it is the whole medical team that is in need of therapy. In the best of all possible worlds, the psychiatrist works consistently with the same medical team. This makes it easier to assess and understand the group dynamics and special problems. The nursing staff, often the personnel who have the most constant and persistent involvement with patients, may be particularly stressed by patients' demands, psychotic illness, or abusive behavior. Providing emotional support for the staff members who are crucial to the patient's treatment can be the most useful aspect of the consultation. Also, explanations about the dynamics of the patient's problems remove the mystery and help the staff to feel more empathic and in control.

Consulting psychiatrists are sometimes asked to assist in the management of patients who are severely mutilated. Gunther (1994) discussed countertransference reactions among staff who work with patients who have had catastrophic injuries—that is, patients who will never be physically normal. The countertransference reactions originate from two sources. The first, "socially universal" factors, involves demands posed by the patients' regression, both physical and psychological. Included in these factors are the patient's misplaced aggression, the thwarting of the staff's narcissistic professional needs, the threat of obligatory identification (exemplified by the phrase "there but for the grace of God go I"), and the staff's disgust and revulsion at the sight of the patient's mutilated body. The second potential source of countertransference reactions, "individualized" factors, reflects the individual residues of the caregivers' own developmental experience (conscious and unconscious) with unresolved issues of dependency, aggression, sexuality, self-esteem, and autonomy. Gunther reported that the staff's unconscious reactions to these factors can lead to negative attitudes that can be heard in staff comments such as "the patient should try harder" or "the patient should complain less," which imply that the patient should dismiss his or her powerful and painful emotions.

On a similar theme, Laatsch and colleagues (1993) addressed the countertransference reactions engendered by working with a multiple amputee patient. The patient, in an effort to assert control over his life, was recalcitrant and noncompliant with rehabilitation. The staff, rather than empathically recognizing the patient's pain and vulnerability, viewed him instead as being ungrateful, unmotivated, provocative, and a threat to their own competence.

These two reports bear vivid testimony to the intensity of feelings that such patients can evoke in those who care for them. Psychiatrists consulting in medical settings of this nature must deal with a multiplicity of emotions that the illnesses and injuries evoke in themselves and in their medical and surgical colleagues. Much of their job as consultant will be to find ways to defuse the staff's feelings of anxiety, rage, humiliation, guilt, and helplessness, thereby avoiding the possibility of psychological abandonment of the patient.

Many illnesses elicit strong feelings in caregivers. Perry and Markowitz (1986), who worked intensively with patients with AIDS-related psychiatric disorders, have written with great clarity about the psychological distresses of these patients and those who treat them. They found that patients with this diagnosis, while still symptom free, frequently prematurely regress to the sick role. It is important for the psychiatrist not to confuse this "state" of dependence with what might otherwise be thought of as a character "trait." This is valuable advice in the evaluation of all patients who are ill, either physically or psychologically.

Perry and Markowitz (1986) have noted that treatment with AIDS patients is most effective when the psychiatrist first lets the patient focus on physical symptoms, taking care not to move too quickly to psychological issues. Patients are greatly helped by clarification, abreaction, and suggestion. Psychiatrists often have to struggle with irrational fears of contagion if the patients touch them or otherwise invade their physical space. An agitated and belligerent AIDS patient wandering the halls of the hospital can arouse intense anxiety in the staff, and there is a need to guard against the resultant tendency to overmedicate. The authors found that it was important not to be premature in suggesting a referral to self-help groups. Early in the illness patients may feel too overwhelmed to consider entering a group. It is a major professional challenge to achieve the best empathic distance, which is neither too close nor too distant. Although Perry and Markowitz directed their comments to work with AIDS patients, their experience can be generalized to work with patients with many other medical disorders.

Forensic Psychiatry

Forensic psychiatry is not exempt from countertransference or the negative intrusion of these unrecognized reactions. Forensic examinations, particularly those that take place over a prolonged length of time, can evoke in the examiner strong feelings of compassion. The natural humanistic desire to be of help, if not consciously monitored, can tempt the psychiatrist to assume the role of therapist—a position that then places the professed objectivity of the forensic examination in jeopardy.

Similarly, treating psychiatrists cannot, without considerable jeopardy, wear two hats—namely, those of therapist and expert witness for their patients. Strasburger and colleagues (1997) described the types of situations in which treating psychiatrists are tempted to step out of their role as therapist into the role of expert witness. When a patient in treatment is sexually assaulted, sustains physical injury in an automobile accident, or experiences another tragedy, it is natural that the treating psychiatrist would have more intimate knowledge of the psychological impact of this event than would an unknown "expert witness." Similarly, in child custody cases, the therapist would usually be most familiar with the patient's parenting skills. Strasburger et al. caution that in these and similar situations, treating psychiatrists need to harness their desire to protect their patients. Attorneys, most of whom are unsophisticated about psychiatry, are generally not aware of the therapeutic problems these situations present. They are correct in their assessment that the treating psychiatrist is obviously the most knowledgeable about the patient, but the attorneys are not necessarily familiar with the potentially damaging effect on the treatment if the therapist assumes the role of expert witness. The authors remind us that there is a clear distinction between the legal process, which is directed toward resolution of disputes, and medicine, which has the goal of healing.

The feelings aroused in the examining psychiatrist will vary depending on the situation under investigation. The study by Long (1994) involved review of the psychiatric examiners' reports in 44 sexual harassment cases. The study revealed some interesting data that can shed light on examiners' feelings in a variety of other types of investigations. Long reviewed the diagnoses made by the plaintiffs' psychiatrists in the sexual harassment cases and, comparing these with those made by the defense psychiatrists, found considerable differences. The plaintiffs' examiners appeared to overemphasize Axis I conditions while minimizing or omitting Axis II conditions. The defense examiners, on the other hand, overemphasized disorders on Axis II while minimizing those on Axis I. Long hypothesized that the plaintiffs' psychiatrists were influenced by a wish to protect the plaintiff, identification with the plaintiff, anger toward the defense, or a desire to affirm sociopolitical beliefs. She purported that the defense examiners were driven by similar wishes but that in their case it was a wish to protect or assist the defendant or an identification with the defendant's anger toward the plaintiff. Long's findings lead us once again to realize the improbability of being completely without bias and the ever-present need to be aware of countertransference distortions.

Reimbursement

It has often been said that of all life's problems, sex and money are the two most psychologically charged and difficult to talk about openly and nondefensively. Some psychiatrists are of the belief that it is the latter, money, that is actually the most difficult—for both therapists and patients.

Issues around patients' payment—discussions about fees, the setting of fees, and dealing with the myriad problems associated with reimbursement—are subjects that have the potential to increase patients' self-understanding, but they are also areas in which there is the potential for distorting countertransferences. One such common reaction is avoidance and denial. Ignoring the fact that a patient is not paying on time, being unusually rigid or strict with a particular patient, and failing to raise or lower fees when circumstances recommend such action are among the signs indicating that the psychiatrist's therapeutic stance is being compromised by countertransference imperatives.

Managed care and third-party payment add an additional dimension to this issue. As described earlier, rare is the psychiatrist who, in the ever-present struggle to deliver high-quality patient care, does not have feelings of frustration and rage at "the system." There is a temptation to tell patients about this frustration or to engage patients in attacks on this outside force. It is not that the realities of administrative problems cannot be discussed with patients, but psychiatrists must be careful not to misuse the treatment situation to ventilate their own anger at authority, deprivation, or other forces. In the process, patients' feelings about authorities, including the therapist, may be missed.

When the Psychiatrist Is Ill

It is one thing to have a patient comment that we are looking tired and ill when we are feeling physically fit, but quite another when, in truth, we are ill. Hearing these words from a patient may be an indication that it is time to deal with our patients about the realities of the problem. What do patients need to know about their doctor's illness? What do they not need to know? When is the psychiatrist acting out some type of countertransference by supplying them with unnecessary information, and when is the provision of information actually useful, enabling the patient to deal more effectively with a real event that at some time is a part of everyone's life history?

It is important to accept that a serious illness can befall us at any age. Counselman and Alonso (1993) remind therapists that they need to realize they are not immune from using all of the familiar mechanisms of defense (denial, reaction formation, and anger) to the therapeutic detriment of their patients.

A patient's experience of her therapist's illness has been written about from an interesting viewpoint by Simon (1990). Simon, herself a therapist, described her reactions when her therapist became ill. These reactions included denial, abandonment, anger, compassion, and concern. This information highlights some of the roads both the treating psychiatrist and the patient must travel in dealing with this difficult situation.

Although patients can, and often must, be told of the realities of the problem, they cannot become caregivers. The therapeutic relationship does not ever include the patient's becoming the caregiver. If the therapist can no longer function as a caregiver, the patient must be told, and told with care and therapeutic compassion as the patient's care is temporarily or permanently transferred to a colleague.

However, responding to such a mixture of transference and reality when it is played off in the real world against a background of one's own physical and emotional vulnerability is a major challenge. Psychiatrists should not try to face this alone. This is the time to talk with a colleague, one who is trusted and respected. There is no escaping the fact that illness has a great potential for every therapist, no matter how insightful, to lose therapeutic perspective. Support from colleagues, supervision of cases, and therapy should all be seriously considered.

Conclusion

Countertransference reactions, both conscious and unconscious, are ever present in the psychiatrist's daily work. They occur in group settings, in the privacy of one's office, in clinics, and in hospitals; with patients who are very sick and others who do not seem so sick; toward referring physicians and ancillary staff; and, ever increasingly, toward third-party payers. Sometimes we are aware of them, and at other times it is those around us who point them out. Although we know that there is a great deal to be learned from these reactions, we often do not welcome their presence. However, it is central to the therapeutic work with our patients for us to look for the presence of these countertransference responses, understand their origins, and use them to further treatment through greater understanding of ourselves and our patients.

References

Adshead G: Psychiatric staff as attachment figures. Understanding management problems in psychiatric services in the light of attachment theory. Br J Psychiatry 172:64–69, 1998

Asnis GM, Kaplan ML, Hundorfean G, et al: Violence and homicidal behaviors in psychiatric disorders. Psychiatr Clin North Am 20: 405–425, 1997

Beitman BD, Chiles J, Carlin A: The pharmacotherapy-psychotherapy triangle: psychiatrist, nonmedical psychotherapist and patient. J Clin Psychiatry 45:458–459, 1984

Busch FN, Gould E: Treatment by a psychotherapist and a psychopharmacologist: transference and countertransference issues. Hospital and Community Psychiatry 44:772–774, 1993

Butterill D, O'Hanlon J, Book H: When the system is the problem, don't blame the patient: problems inherent in the interdisciplinary inpatient team. Can J Psychiatry 37:168–172, 1992

Colson DB, Allen JG, Coyne L, et al: An anatomy of countertransference: staff reactions to difficult psychiatric hospital patients. Hospital and Community Psychiatry 37:923–928, 1986

Counselman EF, Alonso A: The ill therapist: therapists' reactions to personal illness and its impact on psychotherapy. Am J Psychother 47:591–602, 1993

Cramer JA, Rosenheck R: Compliance with medication regimens for mental and physical disorders. Psychiatr Serv 49:196–201, 1998

Dubin WR: The role of fantasies, countertransference, and psychological defenses in patient violence. Hospital and Community Psychiatry 40:1280–1283, 1989

Dubin WR, Wilson SJ, Mercer C: Assaults against psychiatrists in outpatient settings. J Clin Psychiatry 49:338–345, 1988

Freud S: The future prospects of psycho-analytic therapy (1910), in The Standard Edition of the Complete Psychological Works of Sigmund Freud, Vol 11. Translated and edited by Strachey J. London, Hogarth Press, 1957, pp 139–152

Gabbard GO: The therapeutic relationship in psychiatric hospital treatment. Bull Menninger Clin 56:4–19, 1992

Gabbard GO, Takahashi T, Davidson J, et al: A psychodynamic perspective on the clinical impact of insurance review. Am J Psychiatry 148:318–323, 1991

Goin MK: Trust me, a therapist's refrain. Journal of Practical Psychiatry and Behavioral Health, March 1998, pp 115–117

Goin MK, Kline F: Countertransference: a neglected subject in clinical supervision. Am J Psychiatry 133:41–44, 1976

Gunther MS: Countertransference issues in staff caregivers who work to rehabilitate catastrophe-injury survivors. Am J Psychother 48:208–220, 1994

Kahn DA: Medication consultation and split treatment during psychotherapy. J Am Acad Psychoanal 19:84–98, 1991

Laatsch L, Rothke S, Burke WE: Countertransference and the multiple amputee patient: pitfalls and opportunities in rehabilitation medicine. Arch Phys Med Rehabil 74:644–648, 1993

Lion JR, Madden DJ, Christopher RL: A violence clinic: three years' experience. Am J Psychiatry 133:432–435, 1976

Long BL: Psychiatric diagnoses in sexual harassment cases. Bull Am Acad Psychiatry Law 22:195–203, 1994

Madden DJ, Lion JR, Penna MW: Assaults on psychiatrists by patients. Am J Psychiatry 133:422–425, 1976

Main T: The ailment. Br J Med Psychol 30:129–145, 1957

Main T: Traditional psychiatric defenses against close encounters with patients. Canadian Psychiatric Association Journal 22:457–466, 1977

Moore B, Fine B (eds): Psychoanalytic Terms and Concepts. New Haven, CT, American Psychoanalytic Association/Yale University Press, 1968

Perry SW, Markowitz J: Psychiatric interventions for AIDS-spectrum disorders. Hospital and Community Psychiatry 37:1001–1006, 1986

Pi EH, Miller H, Rosenberg MR, et al: Therapeutic effects of psychiatric hospitalization. Journal of Psychiatric Treatment and Evaluation 5:135–142, 1983

Plutnick R, Conte HR, Karasu TB: Critical incidents in psychotherapy. Am J Psychother 48:75–84, 1994

Simon JC: A patient-therapist's reaction to her therapist's serious illness. Am J Psychother 44:590–597, 1990

Steadman HJ, Mulvey EP, Monahan J, et al: Violence by people discharged from acute psychiatric inpatient facilities and by others in the same neighborhoods. Arch Gen Psychiatry 55:393–402, 1998

Strasburger LH, Gutheil TG, Brodsky A: On wearing two hats: role conflict in serving as both psychotherapist and expert witness. Am J Psychiatry 154:448–456, 1997

Swanson JW, Holzer CE, Ganju VK, et al: Violence and psychiatric disorder in the community: evidence from the Epidemiologic Catchment Area surveys. Hospital and Community Psychiatry 41: 761–770, 1990

Swartz MS, Swanson JW, Hiday V, et al: Violence and severe mental illness: the effects of substance abuse and nonadherence to medication. Am J Psychiatry 155:226–231, 1998

Tyson RL: Countertransference evolution in theory and practice. J Am Psychoanal Assoc 34:251–274, 1986

Chapter 4

Countertransference in the Treatment of the Antisocial Patient

John R. Lion, M.D.

In his review of the treatment of antisocial personality disorder, Meloy (1995) summarized a variety of countertransference responses commonly encountered in practice. These include devaluation or condemnation of the patient (Symington 1980) and the illusion that there exists a treatment alliance with him (Gerstley et al. 1989). Helplessness and loss of professional identity (Bursten 1973) may arise as the clinician senses the limited gains possible in therapeutic work. Kindled by anxiety, denial of the patient's harmfulness or danger may also occur (Lion 1978). This chapter explores in greater depth the nature and range of countertransference sentiments in the treatment of antisocial patients.

General Issues in the Countertransference

The clinician confronting a patient with an antisocial or severely narcissistic personality is apt to experience a variety of feelings, ranging from outrage and condescension to admiration and envy. These polarities of evoked countertransference sentiments are complex and shifting and often come as a surprise to the novice practitioner who is more attuned to the "introverted" symptoms whereby patients suffer, are dysphoric or overtly despondent, and display guilt and shame. An exception, perhaps, to this paradigm is the appearance of a flagrantly manic patient or a patient who utilizes extreme projection in the service of a persecutory delusion; but even with these patients, the pathology is so rampant and obvious that sympathy is traditionally the elicited response or the clinician manifestly sees the patient as ill and in need of therapy, hospitalization, or medication.

Patients with antisocial personalities conjure up different affective responses: the desire to make the patient penitent; fear for physical safety; retribution; and even vengeance. To see a murderer or rapist in an incarceration setting is an entirely different clinical experience than, say, to confront a toxic alcoholic or schizophrenic patient who is brought by the police into the emergency room in need of acute intervention. Indeed, the setting itself defines a portion of the countertransference response. Hospitals are places of healing, whereas prisons are primarily for vindictiveness and warehousing. A forensic facility, although a hybrid entity, still has all the ambience of a fortress and is often managed by correctional authorities rather than the state's mental health administration. Many clinicians who begin to spend time in a prison hospital often experience fatigue and a feeling of hopelessness. After all, how can mankind be so bad and deranged at the same time? And how can one possibly tell true suffering from malingering?

Part of the dichotomy of response between "normal" psychiatric patients and those with extremely negative or aggressive character psychopathology lies in the problem of clinician exposure. Few formal residency programs officially rotate students through jails or prisons or forensic facilities, preferring instead to isolate residents from these harsh realities where bad and mad so powerfully intersect. Yet it is only here that a novice therapist can begin to grapple with the elements of manipulation and deceit and to confront the natures of evil and illness. Surrounded by bars and gates, sally ports and hostile guards behind thick glass windows, and the ever-present aura of danger, a resident has no choice but to somehow incorporate criminality into a psychic schema of mental illness and psychological disability. How else can he reconcile the young schizophrenic man who kills his parents? or the delusional bomber? or the recidivistic pedophilic individual? Without a milieu in which to understand these behaviors, clinicians become hopelessly lost, jaded, and frightened by the massive behavioral deviancies that confront them.

Mistrust and Skepticism

An additional problem evoked by seeing antisocial and severely psychopathic patients is the issue of gullibility and naïveté. Most who chose the profession of psychiatry manifestly believe what patients relate to them and come to cherish the values or belief systems of even those patients who might be temporarily psychotic. Yet patients with antisocial personalities lie and distort; they are not to be believed, or if they are believed, it is only with enormous skepticism and challenge. This posture pits the doctor against the patient, as if the former were a policeman attempting to break down the alibi of the accused. Mistrust, suspicion, and wariness are all strong countertransference elements swirling out of work with offender populations, and these elements are quite contrary to the innate trust that characterizes work with neurotic patients seen in an office in a suburban setting. Allied to this is the phenomenon of being "used" or exploited by the antisocial patient, who is always far more skilled at "conning" than any therapist. Chagrin and a sense of being made to look foolish are recurring themes in working with antisocial populations. In time, a hardening process usually occurs whereby the therapist becomes more highly circumspect about what any criminal tells him; but this toughening is quite contrary to the softer and gentler faith that is found in a private office setting, where confrontations are made with style and grace. The famous forensic psychiatrist Manfred Guttmacher typically advised forensic psychiatrists to spend some of their professional time doing conventional office psychotherapy so that they would be less cynical about mankind and more respectful toward and hopeful about conventional psychiatric treatment.

Incarcerated settings pose countertransference problems for both beginning therapists and seasoned clinicians. One large problem is that of mistrust, and it is axiomatic that a prisoner or detainee will not embrace any agent of the institution or even one who has ostensibly been sent specifically to help him. Further, many prisoners do not tell the truth, thus testing the evaluator. The effects here are corrosive, for the clinician is apt to emerge from an interview doubting the data and seeing the patient not as frightened or wary but as corrupt. The proper stance once again is midpoint: to see part truth and part deception and to understand that skepticism is a necessary ingredient of all evaluations conducted under duress. In a private office setting, such skepticism is rarely as rampant. But there is an opposite facet to skepticism, and that is to see a patient as "wronged" and falsely accused or punished. This commonly occurs with juvenile offenders or alleged child molesters who are characterologically passive and more dependent and who espouse an air of complete innocence. With such a "reasonable" patient who appears bewildered about his incarceration, it is incumbent on the clinician to read the chart first lest he be fooled. Many antisocial men (or women) are dangerous, and the devaluation of danger is a common countertransference reaction. It is based partly on denial, partly on the fact that the clinician can dismiss the case and leave the institution at the end of the day, and partly on how the clinician himself sees the world at large. Some clinicians have taken part in adversity via their family, divorce, economic difficulties, or personal traumas. Others have been relatively untouched by such events and may have blind spots when it comes to perceiving evil. It is not uncommon for novice clinicians to be overwhelmed by the magnitude of psychopathology within a prison setting. Crowding, the lack of any meaningful privacy, a harsh physical plant, and a pervasive aura of crisis can create anxiety. Noise levels in prisons are high, and profanity is ubiquitous; these conditions also heighten tension. Incompletely inured to constant danger of escape and personal injury, guards and prison officials adopt a posture of disdain that cannot help but have an impact on the sensitivities of the psychiatrist.

Reactions to Accounts of Violence

Western culture glamorizes violence in film, and implicit admiration of violence is no less an occurrence in the psychic response to criminals who have engaged in brutal or sensational crimes. Psychiatrists evaluating these individuals may tend to brag about the experience and find themselves fascinated with the sadistic elements of the crime—the ability to kill, or kill in a detached way, or harm others. Many clinicians are personally quite inhibited in their expression of aggression and may thus come to almost stand in awe of those who can nakedly show their rages. This countertransference reaction of fascination or even enjoyment at hearing of the violent exploits of patients poses problems in many areas, including an appreciation of the patient's predatoriness, his risk to society, and the extent of his psychosocial deprivation and lack of remorse. An opposite reaction may also occur—namely, the clinician encountering a patient who has committed a brutal crime may be so appalled at the enormity of the crime that he cuts short the anamnesis, either out of revulsion or fright. Women hearing about violent rapes may find themselves too upset to acquire a meaningful history. Some male therapists are wholly intolerant of hearing about aggressive pedophilia, while sexual murders or lust crimes may conjure up raw repulsion that literally shuts down the mind of the listener.

The solution to the polarity of evoked reactions encountered in work with these patients is good supervision by a clinician seasoned in understanding the complex phenomenology of crime. Unfortunately, too often students, residents, and even junior faculty are sent to a jail or prison without any formal review process at all, as if the patients in such facilities lacked the dignity required for an ordinary supervisory experience. Generally speaking, the more heinous the crime, the greater the need for clinical discussion to tease apart psychodynamics from countertransference. Another useful tactic for clinicians encountering the world of crime and antisocial propensities is to join an organization such as the American Academy of Psychiatry and the Law. Members of this group, composed of a mix of practitioners and therapists and those interested in social and sexual psychopathology, serve as role models for the clinician grappling to find a place in the world for both mad and bad persons.

The Background of the Clinician

Clinicians vary considerably in their attitude toward aggression. Some are from backgrounds wholly intolerant of violence and consciously embrace psychiatry for its cognitive components and lack of adverse behaviors. They may choose psychoanalysis, child psychiatry, or psychopharmacology as a means of avoiding behavioral confrontation. When such confrontation does occur, such as on an inpatient service where a patient requires restraint or seclusion, the resident may find himself withdrawing from assistance, support, or even discussion. Conversely, some trainees relish confrontation and may actually become more statistically at risk for assault and threats. Some clinicians can be subtly provocative, whereas others can be so passive that they evoke threats or violence merely as a function of their own helpless demeanor.

Particularly brutal crimes with sexual components, disfigurement, and mutilation, whether committed by sane or insane persons, engender unique affects. There may be "fascination" with the macabre nature of the act, or an inability on the part of the evaluator to view photographs of the crime scene. Numbing can occur, manifested by a curious detachment on the part of the clinician as he attempts to gather specific details about the offense. Some clinicians wrestle with strong punitive emotions and simply wish the perpetrator executed without any attempt to understand the dynamics of the crime. Dread, fear, and even excitement may occur in the face of a notorious crime that the doctor has been called on to evaluate. The clinician should attempt in some way to understand how his upbringing and how parent and authority figures shaped his attitude toward disobedience. Was the show of anger in the family allowed or punished? Was physical anger tolerated?

Training Issues: The Resident as the Victim of Violence

Violence is taught about less than its counterpart, depression. Whereas depression and suicide are traditional academic subjects in residency training programs to which much attention is devoted, violence has always been a stepchild entity. It has been estimated that for every didactic hour spent on aggression and violence, there is much more time spent teaching about depression (American Psychiatric Association 1993). Thus, residents come to learn very late about treatment strategies for managing aggression. Worse, they are usually functionally exempt from handling violent patients who require "takedowns" or restraint and seclusion, all interventions traditionally handled by nursing staff. As a result of being exempted from "combat" operations, clinicians rarely have skills in self-protection and thus are easily immobilized when personally threatened or assaulted. This cannot help but exert an effect on the nature of the countertransference, often converting it to fear, alarm, and avoidance rather than a sense of mastery.

Manifestations of this can be seen when a resident or clinician is threatened (Lion 1995). When uncomfortable with violence, the clinician utilizes denial in dealing with the threat, often minimizing it altogether even when it constitutes an actual hazard to life (Lion and Herschler 1998). In such cases, the clinician may seek consultation only after a long interval has elapsed and the threat has escalated beyond what even denial will support.

Since assaults are not uncommon within psychiatric facilities (American Psychiatric Association 1993; Ladds and Lion 1997), countertransference elements must continually be monitored as crucial parameters of the milieu. Thus, attention must be paid to whether the clinician likes or dislikes the patient and is covertly frightened of him and hence avoidant of confrontation. How the therapist sets limits and says no to certain behaviors is crucial and often based on anger and frustration; this is particularly apt to be the case with highly provocative adolescents. It is permissible—indeed, often therapeutic—for a clinician to admit to his fear of a patient. Patients who seek to distance others do so until the desired effect is achieved. By pointing out to the patient that he is already perceived as dangerous, further escalation can be prevented. But the therapist must be mindful of how he feels about the patient to begin with. Fantasies about the patient are important. Is this someone the clinician actively thinks about? Has he ever feared the patient might come to his home? Has he had angry thoughts about him or wanted to be able to protect himself from the patient by, say, purchasing a weapon?

Narcissism

More subtle countertransference reactions to antisocial personalities and psychopathy can reflect themselves in a deep intrigue in narcissism, entitlement, grandiosity, and the other psychopathologic elements of disordered conscience. The "thrill" of learning about the skillful deceptions of patients who, for example, have embezzled large sums of money can blunt the clinician to an appreciation of consciencelessness and defective superego processes. It is easy to become captivated by a good psychopath and to sit by in rapture as he describes his methodology. Even admiration can be evoked within the therapist, who, after all, struggles with much smaller intrapsychic issues of right and wrong and who is often burdened by his own sense of guilt and contrition. In areas of sexual acting out, this principle plays a role as well when the psychiatrist is confronted with promiscuity and infidelity, particularly if his own relationships are threatened at the same point in time. Thus, the therapist may find himself too permissive, too forgiving, too encouraging of "exploratory" behaviors, and insufficiently challenging and limit setting.

Political figures and prominent men and women seeking treatment evoke particularly difficult countertransferences. Some, such as politicians, skirt many edges of propriety and brag openly or quietly about their victories, strategies, or cunning. Here, the clinician is tested in terms of values, morals, and his own sense of right and wrong. The tone of listening itself assumes importance. If there is a hungry and eager desire to hear about an exploit, it conveys one message. A more subdued posture conveys some degree of doubt that may be useful in pivoting the discussion to larger issues of what is proper and improper behavior.

Drug Abuse and Countertransference

Therapeutic permissiveness also plays a role in the confrontation of behaviors such as drinking, driving and drinking, and drug use. Therapists who have personally endured difficulties with abstinence may be harsher and more confrontational, whereas therapists for whom illicit substance abuse is a mere abstract concept rather than a destructive reality can easily shrug away such behaviors in the patients they treat. But even here, the therapist treads a fine line between harsh and outspoken criticism and censure and passive acquiescence to the patient's actions. There is room for confrontation, and the clinician's demeanor can be one of kindness even though he disapproves of a behavior. Perhaps this "countertransference" amalgam forms the most difficult therapeutic task of all—the one of accepting the patient while disapproving of the behavior. Even in prison work with the very worst of offenders, the stance must be one of conveyed human respect.

It may be tempting to view all behavior as derived from chemical abuse and to overlook character pathology. This countertransference response of seeing a patient as an "alcoholic" or a "drug abuser" exempts him from responsibility and change and oversimplifies treatment. While more blatant and toxic behaviors may cease with abstinence or detoxification, traits such as entitlement and exploitativeness may surface.

Antisocial Women

The countertransference response to women with antisocial personalities often depends on the nature of the crime. If the crime has been defensive in nature, sympathy may be the major reaction in the evaluator. The world of crime is largely male, and it is often forgotten that some female felons may be exceedingly dangerous. Here, attractiveness and other aspects of femininity can blind the clinician to violence and ruthlessness. Or the female patient can espouse a stance of helplessness and victimhood, as if she were merely an accomplice to a man, rather than the principal perpetrator of a crime. Some white-collar crimes committed by older women defy easy scrutiny, particularly when the woman is more "grandmotherly" or presents with a kindly facade that detracts from an appreciation of willfulness and purpose. Seductiveness is a hazard, and the male clinician entering a largely female ward or prison must appreciate the inherent vulnerability of the situation: he will be flattered, admired, sought out, and more easily manipulated. The opposite is true for female clinicians working in largely male settings; namely, they are ready targets for sexual attention. Some find the verbal harassment and joking intolerable.

Identification can occur in cases of domestic abuse in which the evaluator can easily picture herself in a similarly charged situation. Some perpetrators of defensive violence evoke sympathetic responses. Others, by virtue of their victimhood, may generate anger in the evaluator.

The Alien Nature of Crime

Many human criminal acts, especially sexually deviant crimes, are often quite difficult to comprehend and require a frame of reference quite alien to that used by the average clinician who makes medical diagnoses. The *Crime Classification Manual* (Douglas et al. 1992), for example, conceptualizes crimes according to motive and method. Thus, there are organized sexual homicide, disorganized sexual homicide, authority killing, erotomania killing, various classifications for rape, and so forth. The classification is completely different from that in the symptom-based *Diagnostic and Statistical Manual of Mental Disorders* (American Psychiatric Association 1994), which the average clinician uses.

Generally speaking, crime nomenclature and clinical terminology are different languages. Criminal depictions are blunt, descriptive, and often more graphic. Clinicians who grapple with offenses such as serial murders, mass murders, or crimes with prominent sadistic elements may find themselves at a loss because they cannot read about these behaviors in typical medical and psychiatric textbooks. They must revert to other sources of knowledge, including forensic texts and journals. Such materials are rarely subscribed to by departments of psychiatry, though some familiarity with such sources can be gleaned by scanning references to articles published in the *Journal of the American Academy of Psychiatry and the Law.* Also, psychiatrists wishing to understand criminality must befriend colleagues in law enforcement and learn something about the nature of police work. This notion may be initially repellent to the average psychiatrist, who sees the unacademic policeman as existing in a pedestrian, black-and-white world. Yet police work is exceedingly sensitive and difficult, and many policemen and policewomen have much to teach about human behavior and clinical intuition.

Case Example

The following case illustrates many of the countertransference elements discussed in this chapter.

> A young clinician undertook to treat an antisocial and narcissistic inpatient. The patient's behavior was a management problem on the ward, and his manipulations were well known to nursing staff. He drank, had drugs brought in, and provocatively disobeyed rules and regulations; for example, his girlfriend was found in his room after hours. The psychiatrist attempted to understand all these behaviors in psychodynamic terms—that is, as rebellion against harsh parental figures. In the process, the clinician was quite forgiving of actions that dismayed nursing staff. Staff attempted to point out the patient's psychopathic style, while the psychiatrist "excused" the behavior as manifestations of narcissistic illness.
>
> A time came when the patient wished to leave the hospital prematurely. Staff were opposed to this and called on the psychiatrist to intervene. The psychiatrist confronted the patient and evoked his anger. The patient became combative and began to assault the psychiatrist. Fortunately, nearby staff intervened and restrained the patient. Upset by this turn of events, the psychiatrist sought supervision, at which time he revealed his own rigid upbringing and his identification with the patient's rebelliousness. Because of his sympathies, the psychiatrist had not fully explored the extent of the patient's hostilities, lack of empathy, and history of violence.

This case highlights the importance of the clinician's background and shows how denial leads to an impaired appreciation of a patient's dangerousness. The result was an overly patient reaction to the patient's defiance and behavior. The psychiatrist was desirous of avoiding a confrontation and the anger that might accompany it. Distrust and skepticism were also avoided in this process, and limit setting on the patient's drug use was not carried out. Had this patient perhaps been in a forensic setting, the psychiatrist might have been better able to assess his antisocial propensities.

References

American Psychiatric Association, Task Force on Clinician Safety: Clinician Safety (Task Force Report 33). Washington, DC, American Psychiatric Association, 1993

American Psychiatric Association: Diagnostic and Statistical Manual of Mental Disorders, 4th Edition. Washington, DC, American Psychiatric Association, 1994

Bursten B: The Manipulator. New Haven, CT, Yale University Press, 1973

Douglas JE, Burgess AW, Burgess AG, et al: Crime Classification Manual. New York, Lexington Books, 1992

Gerstley L, McLellan T, Alterman A, et al: Ability to form an alliance with the therapist: a possible marker of prognosis for patients with antisocial personality disorder. Am J Psychiatry 146:508–512, 1989

Ladds B, Lion JR: Severe assaults and homicide within medical institutions: epidemiological considerations, in Hospital Security for Health Professionals. Edited by Lion JR, Dubin WR, Futrell D. Chicago, IL, American Hospital Association, 1997, pp 15–24

Lion JR: Outpatient treatment of psychopaths, in The Psychopath: A Comprehensive Study of Antisocial Disorders and Behaviors. Edited by Reid W. New York, Brunner/Mazel, 1978, pp 286–300

Lion JR: Threats against clinicians, in Clinician Safety in Psychiatric Practice. Edited by Eichelman BS, Hartwig AC. Washington, DC, American Psychiatric Press, 1995, pp 43–52

Lion JR, Herschler J: The stalking of clinicians by their patients, in The Psychology of Stalking: Clinical and Forensic Perspectives. Edited by Meloy JR. New York, Academic Press, 1998, pp 165–173

Meloy JR: Antisocial personality disorder, in Treatments of Psychiatric Disorders, 2nd Edition, Vol 2. Gabbard GO, Editor in Chief. Washington, DC, American Psychiatric Press, 1995, pp 2273–2290

Symington N: The response aroused by the psychopath. International Review of Psychoanalysis 7:291–298, 1980

Chapter 5

Countertransference and Assisted Suicide

Francis T. Varghese, M.B.B.S., F.R.A.N.Z.C.P., and Brian Kelly, B.Med., Ph.D., F.R.A.N.Z.C.P.

The role of a doctor in assisting a patient to commit suicide or in taking some other part in the termination of life is complex in the breadth of social, ethical, and psychological implications. There is a tendency to reduce this complexity to discussions about individual rights and legal issues. The underlying dilemma was highlighted by Annas (1993) in his comment that "[d]iscussions of assisted suicide . . . are all symptoms of the problem modern medicine has with dying rather than the solution" (p. 1573). In community, legal, and medical debate on these issues, little attention has been paid to the role of the doctor-patient relationship in end-of-life decisions. Indeed, the impact and meaning of the request for assisted suicide with reference to transference and countertransference in the doctor-patient relationship have not been addressed. This lack of attention to these issues emphasizes the need for research to help us understand the motivation for patient requests for euthanasia and the context of these requests within the doctor-patient relationship. However, there has been relatively little research focusing on dying patients and their doctors regarding such critical issues (Severson 1997). Much more attention has been paid to documenting the attitudes of doctors and the community to euthanasia and end-of-life decisions, as if the issue could be laid to rest by results of opinion polls (Kuhse et al. 1997).

In this chapter, we define euthanasia after Moulin and colleagues (1994) as deliberate actions taken with the intention of ending the patient's life and either assisted or carried out by a health professional, actions in which the death of the patient is the goal. In our opinion, this definition includes physician-assisted suicide, since both euthanasia and physician-assisted suicide involve actions by the doctor with the intention of ending the patient's life. Whether the doctor administers the drug or the patient self-administers the drug provided by the doctor is irrelevant clinically since the intention is the same, although there may be subtle legal differences.

The wish of a patient for an assisted death or euthanasia needs to be evaluated within a broad context that includes the interpersonal, social, and cultural factors that can influence the suffering, concerns, and decision making of the patient. Central to this context is the nature of the relationship between patient and doctor, whether or not one uses the transference-countertransference model to describe the therapeutic frame that defines the medical consultation.

The public debate on euthanasia has focused narrowly on the patient's right to personal choice for death and its timing, and yet, as Miles (1994) has argued, the personal choice for hastened death is formed by interpersonal and social forces shaping the patient's appraisal of his or her illness and situation. The doctor-patient relationship is only one such force but is nevertheless critical in influencing how patients perceive their situation, attribute meaning to it, and make the decision whether to seek assistance to die. The debate in both the professional medical press and the community has generally underestimated the important role of the relationship of the patient to his or her doctor and other health care staff in the issues of adaptation to illness and end-of-life decisions (Ganzini and Lee 1997; Miles 1994; Zalcberg and Buchanan 1997).

Although much has been said of the "right to die," Muskin (1998) has argued that "[n]ot discussing a patient's motivation (for assisted suicide) is the real violation of his or her rights" (p. 327). Legal and ethical debates about euthanasia concentrate on the notion of "rational" decision making, the possible exclusion of major psychiatric disorder at the time, and determination of "competency" to make decisions. These issues are less important at the clinical level than understanding the nature and degree of suffering for patients with terminal illness and the ways in which psychological and social factors influence decision making in this setting (Chochinov and Wilson 1995).

An empathic gap can exist between doctors and some of their patients on the basis of gender, class, culture, and age, among other things. Because in most societies the large majority of doctors come from particular socioeconomic groups, some disadvantaged groups are rendered particularly vulnerable. The cultural context of the dominant ethical and legal debate (including the assumption of the overriding ethical status of individual autonomy), along with the cultural context and meaning of the care of the dying, of illness, and of suffering, also needs to be acknowledged (Glick 1997; Kleinman 1995). Holland (1991) points out that "the current emotional debate about the appropriate role of physician-assisted suicide for cancer patients who wish to die has been based far too long on personal beliefs and personal bias and far too little on objective observations."

In this chapter we discuss evidence emerging from a range of research in clinical populations concerning terminally ill patients, end-of-life and other treatment decisions by medically ill patients, and the impact of care of the dying patient on the treating doctor. The research provides an empirical basis for the discussion that follows, addressing the broader psychodynamic issues, including the role of countertransference and projective identification, in order to highlight important clinical factors that have been relatively neglected to date in this area (Kelly and Varghese 1996). Indeed, empirically based research demonstrates the complexity of the situation faced by terminally ill patients and contradicts many popular misconceptions.

Suicide and "Rational" Suicide in the Terminally Ill

It is frequently assumed that patients who have been diagnosed with cancer and other severe physical illness will consider suicide and, moreover, that suicide is "rational" in cases of severe illness in which no treatment is available. In fact, the available evidence indicates that even though suicide risk may be increased in cancer patients, suicide accounts for only a small minority of deaths in this population (Allebeck and Bolund 1991; Breitbart 1990; Heitanen and Lonnqvist 1991; Storm et al. 1992). When suicide and attempted suicide do occur in cancer patients, they are closely associated with major psychiatric disorders, particularly depression (Breitbart 1990). The association with psychiatric disorder also applies to the wish to die in other terminally ill patients (Brown et al. 1986; Chochinov et al. 1995). Furthermore, depression and psychological symptoms are difficult to detect and frequently underdiagnosed and undertreated, particularly in patients with chronic physical illness or in the terminally ill (Conwell and Caine 1991; Hendin and Klerman 1993), casting further doubt on the assessment of "rational" suicide in the terminally ill. Such underdiagnosis and undertreatment of psychiatric illness may reflect particular emotional reactions in doctors to the terminally ill, representing a countertransference issue rather than a question of diagnostic acumen alone. Doctors treating terminally ill patients tend to consider the patient's mood state as "normal" on the assumption that they would feel the same if they were in a similar situation (Miles 1994), a situation of pseudoempathy. Significant doubt must be cast on the concept of rational suicide in patients with terminal illness and on efforts to normalize suicide and suicidal ideation in this group (Conwell and Caine 1991).

The severity of physical illness may be of less significance in the patient's decision to end life, or indeed in making other treatment decisions, than the basic adaptive pattern of the individual and the impact of this on the patient's response and the responses of those around him or her (Baile et al. 1993). The importance of the basic adaptive pattern of the individual and of its impact is borne out in studies of correlates of the wish to die and suicidal ideation in patients with medical illness (Breitbart et al. 1996; Chochinov et al. 1995). It also emerges in studies of "medically assisted death" among individuals with AIDS (Bindels et al. 1996), studies of patients' evaluations of quality of life and disability (Rothwell et al. 1997; Uhlmann and Pearlman 1991), and studies of patients with end-stage renal failure who elect to die by withdrawal of dialysis (Hirsch 1989).

Suicidal ideation is not predicted by the severity of disease or objective indices of quality of life in medically ill patients (Breitbart et al. 1996; Fogel and Mor 1993); nor does it seem to be the normal reaction of a dying individual (Seigel 1982). This highlights the need for physicians to fully understand the clinical correlates of the wish to hasten the death in the terminally ill so as to fully appreciate the factors that promote understanding of the total context of the request for assisted suicide from terminally ill patients.

In a study involving more than 300 men with AIDS, having an "interest" in physician-assisted suicide was predicted by high levels of psychological distress and the experience of terminal illness of a friend or relative and by a perception of lower levels of social support. There was no significant association between interest in assisted suicide and severity of the disease (Breitbart et al. 1996). Chochinov and colleagues (1995) examined the desire for death in a group of more than 100 terminally ill cancer patients. The authors found that only 8.5% had an enduring and clinically significant desire for death, and of these the diagnostic criteria for major depression were fulfilled in 59%, compared with 8% of those without a stated desire for death. Pain, lower levels of family support, and depression were significantly associated with the desire for death. An important finding here is that the desire for death was temporally unstable, thus raising concern about assisting in a patient's requested suicide at any particular point in the disease. This also emphasizes the dangers in evaluating a request for assisted suicide in the absence of a relationship with the patient over a significant period of time and highlights particularly the difficulties in assessments in which "competence" is the only issue considered. In one survey, whereas only 6% of 321 Oregon psychiatrists were "very confident" in conducting a psychiatric assessment with respect to physician-assisted suicide, 66% supported physician-assisted suicide as a medical treatment option (Ganzini et al. 1996). It seems that the confidence of psychiatrists in the assessment of physician-assisted suicide is not matched by their beliefs in supporting physician-assisted suicide.

In an important study of suicides by cancer patients in Finland (Heitanen and Lonnqvist 1991), it was found that inadequate symptomatic treatment, failure to pay sufficient attention to the patient's psychological needs, and a lack of a doctor with a long-term responsibility for treatment were key issues associated with suicide in this group. The authors emphasized the patients' feelings of abandonment and rejection that can occur when the doctor-patient relationship is brought to an end because of the lack of curative treatment. They also highlight that all of these factors contribute to a patient's perception that illness and dependency have become intolerable.

Several issues contribute to the request for assisted suicide or euthanasia. Cherny and colleagues (1994a, 1994b) include among these issues uncontrolled physical symptoms, unrecognized depression or anxiety, unaddressed existential distress, and unrecognized and unaddressed family member and health care provider fatigue. To this can be added the factors associated with suicide among cancer patients outlined by Breitbart (1993), such as loss of control and helplessness, depression and hopelessness, delirium (especially mild delirium with diminished impulse control in an already depressed patient), preexisting psychopathology, suicide history (including the history of attempted suicide and suicides by family members), chronicity of illness, and withdrawal from the patient by family and doctors.

In a study of 93 cancer patients who had attempted suicide, Breitbart (1987) found that hopelessness was a key factor in the attempted suicide. The other important factor was the patient's being offered no further treatment and no further contact with the health system, such as was found in the study by Heitanen and Lonnqvist (1991). Breitbart's finding is echoed in the study by Owen and colleagues (1994) of 102 cancer patients; the authors found that hopelessness and lack of social support were important in bringing about a wish for suicide or euthanasia.

Other reports have indicated that the experience of pain from cancer is indirectly related to suicidal ideation and the wish to die, with levels of depression, hopelessness, and perceived family support being important mediating variables (Chochinov and Wilson 1995; Chochinov et al. 1995). The patient's perception of poor pain relief has been found to be more closely associated with suicidal ideation, and this suggests that a perception of inadequate pain relief may have more to do with hopelessness, since pain intensity itself was not found to be a significantly correlating factor (Breitbart 1990). This suggestion is consistent with the findings linking suicidal ideation with levels of hopelessness in terminally ill patients (Chochinov et al. 1998).

While suicide in patients with HIV / AIDS has been reported to be associated with psychiatric disorder (Marzuk et al. 1988), it has also been shown that suicide is related not to severity of illness or prognosis but to factors such as lack of social support and past psychiatric illness (O'Dowd et al. 1993; Rajs and Fugelstad 1992; Rundell et al. 1992). The clinically important finding is that among people with HIV infection, suicidal ideation occurs soon after the diagnosis rather than later, when the patient's illness is indeed terminal (O'Dowd et al. 1993; Rundell et al. 1992). Many psychological and social factors have a bearing on levels of suicidal ideation independent of disease severity in HIV infection (Kelly et al. 1998).

The strong advocacy for euthanasia and assisted suicide for people suffering from the consequences of HIV infection on the part of HIV advocacy groups is worth exploring. It seems paradoxical that the advocates for HIV-infected persons, who have had a powerful and crucial role in breaking down public misperceptions and unwarranted fear about HIV infection, should be advocates for euthanasia for those whom they regard as their constituency, thus inadvertently affirming the conscious or unconscious wishes of an arguably prejudiced community that HIV-infected persons were dead. Could compassion fatigue be an issue here? We suggest that social and cultural reactions to illness and death in general, and perhaps HIV infection in particular, need to be considered.

The findings outlined above concerning suicide and suicidal ideation link with evidence concerning "quality of life" evaluation of patients with cancer or chronic physical illness and elderly patients and their perceptions of the disability imposed by disease and of their treatment choices, which may vary significantly from their doctors' perceptions (Rothwell et al. 1997; Slevin et al. 1990; Uhlmann and Pearlman 1991). Such studies suggest that clinicians frequently use "quality of life" judgments in overestimating their own wish for treatment cessation or for nonactive treatment. The ill-defined and overused concept of "quality of life" is regularly brought to bear in support of assisted suicide decisions (Gaita 1995).

The subjective evaluation by a doctor of the patient's "quality of life" and the role of such an evaluation in making end-of-life decisions of themselves raise significant countertransference issues. Inaccurately putting oneself "in the patient's shoes" in order to make clinical decisions and evaluations of quality of life leaves the patient vulnerable to the doctor's personal and unrecognized issues concerning illness, death, and disability. Hendin (1994) argues that doctors may presume that decisions can be based on what they themselves would wish if they were in the patient's situation, bringing the doctor-patient relationship to a new dimension: the wishes of the doctor for the patient are presumed to be identical to those of the patient. This emphasizes the importance of addressing countertransference issues before concluding that what one experiences with the dying patient is indeed empathy rather than countertransference enactment (Adler 1994).

The Interpersonal Context in the Desire for Death

The research outlined in the previous section suggests that there is a lot more to patients' wishes to kill themselves or to seek assisted suicide than a "rational" response to the illness, or indeed the presence of concurrent psychiatric morbidity. What stands out in terminally ill patients is the role of key relationships, social support, and the patient's social environment, including the patient's relationship with the doctor that underlines the patient's decision with respect to end of life.

The needs and responses of the family of the dying patient are important to consider in this regard (Kissane et al. 1994a, 1994b). Cherny and colleagues (1994a) have used the term *empathic distress* to describe the perception by the patient of the distress of family and health care providers that further compounds the patient's distress and thus contributes to the conclusion that ongoing existence only constitutes a burden to others. They have used the term *family fatigue* to describe a factor that may contribute to the request by the patient for assisted death. Anticipated grief, withdrawal of the family from the patient, unrelieved and overriding concerns for the patient's comfort, and a preoccupying need to be with the patient at the time of death all contribute to such fatigue.

We suggest that similar factors could apply to the doctor-patient relationship in the context of the dying patient, with such factors leading to "doctor fatigue." Attending to a dying patient can be among the most stressful experiences in medicine as one confronts powerlessness and hopelessness and the complex emotional responses of the dying patient and of his or her family (Miles 1994; Muskin 1998). This is particularly the case when there is a long-term relationship with the patient. In addition to the resulting anticipatory grief that may be experienced, there is the immediacy of confrontation with the suffering of patients and their families and the apparent futility of medical interventions aimed at cure of disease. The doctor can be a key agent in the overall system of relationships and influences that surrounds the patient, and is as much a participant as an observer in assessing the emotional responses of this system.

In this context, the findings from research concerning the reasons for euthanasia as reported by doctors who have participated in euthanasia are of interest. In a nationwide survey of medical practitioners conducted in the Netherlands (van der Maas et al. 1991), the reasons given by the physicians for the request for suicide included "loss of dignity" (57%), pain (46%), "unworthy dying" (46%), being dependent on others (33%), and "tiredness of life" (23%). However, in only 10 of 187 cases was pain the sole reason for the assisted suicide. Curiously, there has been very little research examining the reason for the request as reported by the patient. The study by van der Maas and colleagues relied on retrospective accounts by the doctors who participated in the deaths of the patients. These doctors may have underreported and failed to detect significant psychological symptoms and potentially remediable patient and family issues, or they may not have reported the difficulties that they as doctors had encountered in managing the patient's illness and distress. The majority of cases of assisted suicide occurred in the patient's home and involved the general practitioner in the setting of a long-term relationship with the patient, whereas fewer cases were reported in institutional settings such as nursing homes (van der Maas et al. 1991).

With the growing emphasis on community-based care of the dying, attention needs to be given to the meaning of such findings. Many factors may contribute to the preponderance of cases arising in the home care setting. The question can be raised whether the absence of professional support and psychodynamic supervision, along with the burden of individual clinical responsibility without the advantages of team-based multidisciplinary care, may adversely affect clinical decision making. In community-based care of individuals with chronic illness and in palliative care, attention needs to be given to the needs of the general practitioner. van der Maas et al. (1991) reported that "many respondents mentioned that an emotional bond is required for euthanasia and this may be one reason why euthanasia was more common in general practice where doctor and patient have often known each other for years and the doctor has shared part of the patient's suffering" (p. 673). They also commented that in their survey of Dutch clinicians, many who had practiced euthanasia indicated that they would be reluctant to do so again. In speculation on the meaning of this, it is important to recognize that many doctors control their aggression through the practice of helping others, and participation in euthanasia may violate the doctor's carefully developed sense of self as a benign and caring figure (Gabbard 1985).

It is clear then that there is ample clinical evidence from studies of patients suffering from terminal illness to indicate that a patient's decision to attempt suicide or to seek assistance in suicide or euthanasia is not a simple matter. The total psychosocial context patients find themselves in plays a crucial role in determining their wishes, and the patient's relationship with the doctor plays a central part as well. There is also evidence to support the view that the difficulties doctors have in dealing with dying patients may influence the patients' appreciation of their situation and their decisions and, indeed, the doctor's decisions. If withdrawal from the patient by the doctor is an influence on the patient's suicidality, it is even more important that doctors understand their feelings about a patient in the clinical situation.

Doctors and Death

It is well recognized that doctors have great difficulty in dealing with death and dying, and, indeed, dealing with terminally ill patients can be emotionally draining for the doctor (Kelly and Varghese 1997). Death anxiety is common among medical practitioners and is likely to affect their attitudes and practices in the care of the dying patient (Viswanathan 1996). Fears of death and illness and of the dependency that may accompany illness, and, indeed, a disgust with disease, may be powerful unconscious motivators for some doctors (Gabbard 1985; Miles 1994). Doctors may have greater difficulty facing their sense of impotence and helplessness when they also carry considerable feelings of responsibility, guilt, and sense of failure if the patient does not recover (Clarke 1981; Gabbard 1995; Miles 1994).

Cassell (1982) has argued that the medicalization of suffering has left doctors ill equipped to address the psychological needs of patients or to identify the source of their suffering and its meaning. Rather, the doctor may seek biological and physical treatments alone. When these fail to provide the solution, doctors may feel there is little left to offer and may withdraw from the patient as a reaction to the feelings of failure and guilt and the confrontation with the limitations of their treatments. Such reactions may inadvertently accentuate the patient's sense of hopelessness, fear of abandonment, and potentially their wish to die (Modestin 1987). The difficulty of facing the patient's anger and disappointment, or the doctor's fear of being the focus of such intense negative emotion, may fuel the doctor's retreat from the patient, promote reaction formation with overinvolvement, or stimulate the development of intense negative feelings toward the patient.

Thomas (1980), as quoted by Annas (1993, p. 1573), has argued that doctors are "as frightened and bewildered by the act of death as anyone else," and Annas (1993) further commented that "[i]t is thus not surprising that many physicians have difficulty talking candidly with dying patients and caring for them." Pellegrino (1993), who argues strongly against the ethical and clinical basis for assisted suicide, asserts that it is often falsely implied that the initiative for physician-assisted suicide is in the patient's hands, when much of the clinical evaluation and provision of means is in the hands of the doctor. He argues that "misdirected compassion in the face of human suffering can be as dangerous as indifference" and that "physicians' evaluation of life and its meaning, the value or non-value of suffering, the kind of life they would find bearable, and the point at which life becomes unbearable cannot fail to influence their decisions" (p. 874). Miles (1994) has described the "emotional disorientation" that the doctor can experience, given the stress of caring for the dying patient, and the impact of this disorientation on the doctor's evaluation of treatments and clinical decisions.

Clearly, caring for the dying patient can be among the most stressful experiences in medicine as one confronts powerlessness and helplessness. The experience is particularly stressful when the doctor has a long-term relationship with the patient, with the resultant grief that may be experienced, and is confronted by the suffering of the patient and family. Despite the impact of this experience, generally little attention has been paid to these issues in medical training (DiMaggio 1993).

Pellegrino (1993), in his discussion of the nature of compassion, argues for the containment of the identification with the patient's suffering (a distorting pseudoempathy or projective identification), stating that "morally weighty as it is, compassion can become maleficent unless it is constrained by principle" (p. 875). Pellegrino also points out, as noted earlier, that "physicians' valuation of life and its meaning, the value or non-value of suffering, the kind of life they would find bearable, and the point at which life becomes unbearable cannot fail to influence their decisions" (p. 874).

Hendin (1994) has commented:

> My own experience has been that many patients and physicians displace many anxieties about death onto the circumstances of dying—pain, dependence, loss of dignity, as well as the unpleas-

> ant side effects resulting from medical treatment, or, for the physician, frustration at not being able to offer a sure cure. Focusing on or becoming enraged at the process distracts from the fear of death itself. Confronting such fear may focus a patient on what he can achieve in whatever life can still offer. (p. 128)

Hendin further notes:

> Patients are not alone in their inability to tolerate situations they cannot control. . . . By deciding when patients die, by making death a medical decision, the physician has the illusion of mastery over the disease and the accompanying feelings of helplessness. (p. 129)

It is often argued that by the doctor's providing what the patients say they want, the decision is independent of any imposition of the doctor's values, a view that underestimates the role of the physician's values in the clinical interaction (Hendin 1994). The doctor's values, opinions on this issue, and countertransference responses may be enacted in his or her behavior and communication with the patient. The way the patient's request for assisted suicide is explored by the doctor and the questions the doctor does or does not pose to the patient are critical here (Hendin 1994; Pellegrino 1993). Hendin (1994) has emphasized that some individuals appear less depressed once they have decided to kill themselves and has argued that the need to maintain control, to make demands on life that cannot be fulfilled in the midst of life's uncertainties, may be a characteristic of suicidal individuals. The role of depression may be underestimated, and the patient's responses to his or her illness may be accepted as "rational" on superficial evaluation in which the psychological meaning of these responses and the defenses of the patient are not explored or understood (Hendin 1994; Seigel 1982). This becomes a particular problem when the anxieties of the patient, as well as the defenses used, resonate with the doctor's own vulnerabilities, such as the need to maintain control. As a consequence, these inflexible demands of the patient are not questioned (Gabbard 1985). The feelings of futility and hopelessness often recognized in the patient may be as much the doctor's dilemma as the patient's. For some doctors, the patient's wish to die may provoke an unrecognized relief to the frustration, helplessness, and, perhaps, guilt and responsibility, because their own distress at the failure of their treatment may distort their responses and judgment (Modestin 1987).

The distress faced by doctors in the task of caring for patients who are dying or have disease such as cancer is well documented (Cherny et al. 1994a, 1994b; Clarke 1981; Ramirez et al. 1995, 1996) and includes frequent feelings of hopelessness, failure, and demoralization. The rates of psychological distress among cancer clinicians and hospital consultants were reported in two studies by Ramirez and colleagues (1995, 1996). The case rate of 27%–28% on the General Health Questionnaire (12 items) found in these studies is similar to the rates reported for many other samples of doctors at all levels of training. The doctors reported that "dealing with the suffering" of their patients was a key stress. A substantial proportion reported inadequate training in communication skills (45%–54%) and management skills (>70%), which was associated with higher levels of distress and greater difficulties in coping with the suffering of patients and others as well as in dealing with other aspects of patient care. Palliative care clinicians reported the lowest rates of stress associated with patients' suffering, a finding perhaps indicative of the benefits of training for those working in palliative care, the emphasis in palliative care on psychological needs of patients and families, and/or the importance of considering the personal characteristics of those who choose a career in this field.

The negative influence of clinical work on oncologists has also been explored by Whippen and Canellos (1991), who found that oncologists experienced high levels of distress and demoralization, with their work having a major impact on their personal and social lives. Contributing factors were a high level of frustration due to limited therapeutic success and the continued exposure to fatal illness.

For general practitioners (Schaerer 1993), the key stresses in the care of a dying patient included the ending of the doctor-patient relationship, coping with feelings of failure and uselessness, awareness of one's own mortality, and feelings of loneliness, sadness, helplessness, and failure. The more personal nature of the relationship seems important in this context.

Given this context of recognized sources of distress for doctors and a perception of insufficient training in critical areas of practice, particularly communication with patients and families (Cantor et al. 1993), it is a matter of concern that physician-assisted suicide and euthanasia are being proposed more strongly than are efforts to understand and address these difficulties in training and clinical experiences. Such support for physician-assisted suicide may be "symptomatic" of the difficulties that doctors themselves highlight as experiencing in treating the terminally ill.

The claim is frequently heard that doctors owe actions such as assisted suicide to patients for whom medicine has failed to offer palliation or cure. The terms "hopelessly ill" (Quill et al. 1992) and "medical failures" (Brody 1992) used to describe dying patients may indicate the discomfort with noncurative treatment and terminal illness within medicine and the perception of death of the patient as a "failure" of medicine. This may be a reaction of the doctor whose patient has an incurable or terminal illness, because the doctor experiences feelings of personal failure, guilt, and responsibility for the patient's illness and disease well beyond any realistic appraisal. Yet such feelings may fuel reactions in the doctor that serve to fend off the discomfort and anxiety that therapeutic failure causes, as the need to feel helpful, to be able to restore function, and to be effective is challenged by the dying patient. Being able to "provide" assisted suicide may become one such response by the doctor to his or her own feelings of futility and failure, but one that is in a form that disguises unacceptable feelings in an attempt to regain a sense of mastery and omnipotence and that has dangerous consequences.

Suicide, it should be remembered, is not a therapy or treatment (Miles 1994), yet it is presented in some literature as having a place in the therapeutic armamentarium, to be used in response to the suffering of the terminally ill (Brody 1992). The doctor may walk an uneasy path between facing the patient's suffering and distress with its many determinants, ideally attempting to maintain empathy and avoiding overidentification (Duckworth et al.

1994), and facing therapeutic limitations in a culture that encourages medical action, therapeutic omnipotence, and technological aspects of medical care. Not surprisingly, some authors have criticized the "medicalization" of suffering, in which doctors feel compelled to provide physical treatments as a solution to suffering rather than understand the personal, interpersonal, and existential issues involved (Cassell 1982). Similarly, the importance of the therapeutic role of the doctor-patient relationship, of the psychotherapeutic aspects of that relationship, and of the role of psychosocial aspects of medical care has been underestimated.

Assessment of Competence and the Therapeutic Frame

In 1995 the Parliament of the Northern Territory in the Commonwealth of Australia enacted the first law anywhere in the world that legally allowed a doctor to give a lethal injection to patients suffering from terminal illness at their request (Ryan and Kaye 1996). Although the practice of assisted suicide or euthanasia had for several years been tolerated in the Netherlands, it technically remained illegal.

Before the Northern Territory law was overturned by the Australian Federal Parliament, four patients had their lives terminated in the Northern Territory, all by the same doctor. Northern Territory law required that the patient requesting euthanasia be examined by a psychiatrist to determine the patient's competency to make such a request; this requirement was designed as a safeguard for patients who might be depressed or suffering from some other mental disorder and who request euthanasia when in other circumstances, or after appropriate treatment of the depression or other mental illness, they might not make such a request (Ryan 1995; Ryan and Kaye 1996). However, little attention was paid in the public debate to the very narrow definition of the process of psychiatric diagnosis and, indeed, the nature of the psychiatrist's or other doctor's relationship with the patient in the clinical interview. In the United States, the Oregon legislation has a similar requirement for the assessment of the patient by a psychiatrist or psychologist in order to determine competency

(Ganzini et al. 1996). It is surprising that little has been written about the meaning of such an assessment in a clinical situation and in the context of the doctor-patient relationship.

The arguments put forward in defense of such legislation assume that doctors in their relationships with patients are essentially benign and will act rationally in the interests of their patients. This position does not take into account the complexities of the relationship, including unconscious and psychodynamic factors that may influence a doctor's responding to a request for euthanasia. The wish to die on the part of the patient may be accompanied by or be a reflection of countertransference wishes on the part of the doctor. Apart from issues of transference and countertransference, a purely legalistic view of the role of the psychiatrist in assessing competency in patients requesting euthanasia in itself undermines the therapeutic frame that allows a doctor to listen to what the patient is saying.

Every psychiatric interview, whether specifically for psychotherapeutic purposes or for the purposes of assessment during a forensic assessment, occurs within a therapeutic frame that limits the actions of both parties and implicitly recognizes that there is a boundary as well as an interpersonal context in the relationship between the doctor and patient (Gutheil and Gabbard 1993). This is not to mystify the doctor-patient relationship, but only to point out that there is a contextual subtext in the relationship that allows the formal contract between the two to function.

The first part of the task of the psychiatrist is to listen to the patient, not just to understand the literal content of what the patient is saying, but also to take into account the context and nature of the relationship (Miles 1994; Muskin 1998). In phenomenological terms, the doctor is operating by two different modes of reasoning and action (Jaspers 1963; Varghese 1988). The first of these is the mode of causal connections, in which the content and meaning of a patient's statements are viewed within the explanatory mode of the natural sciences. The other mode is what Jaspers terms "the psychology of meaningful connections," in which the principal way of operating is that of bringing understanding to a patient's life history and current predicament using empathy as a tool. In the setting of a dying patient's request, both modes of understanding are essential, but the legal framework acknowledges and allows only the first. The richness of meaningful connections that illuminate the totality of the patient's existence and predicament is lost when the psychiatrist is forced into the narrow issue of determining competence.

The context in which a patient requests euthanasia or assisted suicide requires examination in the same way as does the context in which a request for other boundary crossing or boundary violation from the doctor is made. Is it possible to examine the context if there is no prohibition against euthanasia or assisted suicide? Although the therapeutic frame in which the doctor and patient operate has many facets, central to its structure are a series of injunctions limiting the doctor's behavior and the requirement that the doctor always act in the interests of the patient rather than his or her own interests. Because the frame has limits, the patient is allowed to say personal and private things to the doctor within an environment known to be safe and that will contain the patient's fears and impulses (Gutheil and Gabbard 1993). In psychotherapy, for example, patients are able to talk to the doctor about their sexual difficulties and their sexual fantasies, including in some cases their sexual fantasies about the doctor, because they know that the relationship is predefined as one that does not allow a sexual relationship to occur between the two (Gabbard 1996). The prohibition is so implicit that it does not have to be stated to the patient beforehand or written in a contract. It is this prohibition that allows patients the freedom to talk about their feelings and concerns (Sandler et al. 1992).

If a patient did request a sexual relationship from his or her doctor, it would not be regarded as an autonomous request but would be examined in the context of the relationship, regardless of which school of therapy the doctor adhered to, if any. So implicit is the prohibition that a doctor, in response to such a request, does not have to tell the patient, "But I must inform you that I am prohibited by the state authorities, the medical board, and my doctors' association from engaging in a sexual relationship with you." Indeed, a doctor who makes such a statement has clearly missed the point of the patient's statement in the total context of the relationship. In spite of the prohibition against a sexual relationship between a doctor and patient, there are still cases in which this boundary is crossed by unethical therapists. When this happens, even if the boundary violation is driven by powerful countertransference forces, no one considers the doctor's transgression justified. A question like "Does the patient really mean it?" or "Is he or she competent to request a sexual relationship?" is meaningless. The very concept of individual autonomy to make decisions about one's life, including sexual behavior, would have no meaning in this context. The therapeutic frame that allows a patient to examine the sexual transference is held together by the existence of the prohibition, and without the prohibition the patient would be deprived of an opportunity to understand his or her feelings and desires in a therapeutic manner.

Miles (1994) has argued that the "constructive taboo" on physician-assisted suicide is important for the therapeutic relationship between the doctor and the terminally ill patient, inasmuch as it prevents actions that are based on the doctor's own fear of dying, thereby providing a landmark amid the complex emotions that arise in the relationship with the patient. The result is a framework that enables the development of "therapeutic insight into a patient's pain, demoralization and depression" (Miles 1994, p. 1787). Thus, such a framework or boundary enables the doctor to better understand the basis and meaning of the patient's suffering, since it creates a secure therapeutic relationship and consequently enables the doctor to be better able to care for the patient.

When a psychiatrist is determining whether the patient requesting euthanasia is competent to do so, what does the removal of the prohibition against participating in killing the patient do to the therapeutic frame? How can a psychiatrist make sense of the patient's wish to die, and indeed to be put to death if the psychiatrist's role is to determine competence, divorced from the context of the patient's statements or their underlying meaning? How can the extent to which the clinical situation affects the feelings of the doctor and the patient for each other be examined when the central question in the doctor's mind is not "What does this patient mean when he requests euthanasia?" or "What is going on within me that has contributed to the patient's making such a request?" or "Is the patient responding to my needs and psychopathology?," all of which are questions a doctor should ask if a patient seeks a boundary violation in the sexual arena, but rather "Does he really mean it?" The very action of the doctor's attempting to assess competence in the absence of the prohibition against killing the patient, even at the patient's request, shatters the therapeutic frame that allows the request to be examined and dealt with therapeutically. Thus, in a situation in which assisted suicide or euthanasia is legalized, the psychiatrist has been asked to stand outside the therapeutic frame that contains the complexities of emotions within the doctor-patient relationship. The patient is also outside the frame that therapeutically contains the patient's love, hate, fears, and destructiveness and is thereby unprotected against the doctor's feelings, whether these be conscious or unconscious.

Countertransference: The Intersubjectivity of the Request for Physician-Assisted Suicide

The patient's request for euthanasia may be more than just a reflection of the patient's individual despair; it may be an indication that others have despaired of the patient or have been perceived by the patient as having experienced such despair. The patient may be saying to the doctor, "I think you are sick of me," "I think you find my illness a burden," "I know you are disgusted with disease and decay," or "I know you would rather spend time with patients you can help than with somebody who is beyond help." When patients request assistance from their relatives in carrying out suicide, or ask their relatives to intervene on their behalf with the doctor, they may be making similar contextual statements to them. Thus, when euthanasia is put forward as "putting an end to misery," we need to ask, "Just whose misery are we talking about?" (Goodwin 1991). In this context, it is worth noting that all of the patients who made public statements about their request for euthanasia in the Northern Territory stated in one way or the other that they could not let their relatives continue to suffer (Commonwealth of Australia 1997).

For every patient who is suffering and in despair, there are a host of other players who have an interest in that suffering's coming to an end for reasons that may be less than altruistic. A strong association between family functioning and individual psychological morbidity, including depression, has been reported in a study conducted in Melbourne, Australia (Kissane et al. 1994a, 1994b). Depression, anxiety, anger, and overall psychological distress interact among family members during palliative care, particularly anger and hostility among offspring. These patterns may be a reflection, in part, of the demands of care, established patterns of family relationships, and family functioning and communication that may directly or indirectly have an impact on the patient's psychological responses and perception of illness. Similar findings have also been reported by Kissane and colleagues (1996) among bereaved families, providing further validity to the systemic models needed to understand the psychological milieu in which the patient and his or her family respond to terminal illness.

Although relatives are legally prohibited from assisting in the death of terminally ill patients, advocates of voluntary euthanasia have argued that doctors should not be prohibited from providing such assistance. Implicit is the assumption that doctors' feelings about their patients are invariably benign. Put another way, this view assumes that the doctor's countertransference is always positive and helpful and can never be negative and destructive. These are dangerous assumptions (Adler 1994; Gabbard 1996; Winnicott 1949). The legal and ethical arguments in favor of euthanasia, which enshrine the principle of individual patient autonomy, fail to address the question that the wish to die on the part of the patient may be accompanied by or a reflection of the wish to kill on the part of the doctor. Although doctors are ethically and legally constrained from acting on their love of or lust for patients, there is very little to stop them acting on their hate of patients, although it may be disguised as love (Gabbard 1996), if the therapeutic frame that allows the relationship between doctor and patient to work is shattered by the legal removal of prohibition.

In the care of the dying patient, the doctor may experience countertransference feelings of impotence and rage toward the patient, triggered by a perception that all his or her therapeutic efforts are thwarted by the patient. Also, if the family of the patient feels exhausted and futile about the patient, in part reflecting a projected aspect of the patient's experience, the doctor may also feel the same way. If the family comes to feel "We wish you would relieve us of this burden," the doctor may also develop similar feelings about the patient, so that the projective identification mechanism may become consistent across the patient's relationships or the external objects in the patient's life.

The general public and advocates of voluntary euthanasia would be taken aback at the suggestion that doctors could feel destructively toward patients to the extent of hate and disgust and that this could influence decisions regarding whether to proceed with a patient's request for assisted suicide. Is the danger of countertransference issues overstated? We contend that apart from doctors who are excessively saintly or those lacking in a capacity for insight and self-reflection, most doctors would confess that in dealing with a large variety of patients, in whatever field of medicine we are in, there are patients we like, patients we dislike, patients whose conditions cause us frustration and despair, and, finally, patients whom we wish we were not troubled by or burdened with. Fortunately, our ethical code demands that regardless of our personal feelings about particular individuals, we are obliged to treat them with the utmost care and consideration and give them the best possible treatment, and indeed to put their interests ahead of our personal interests or feelings. It is important for doctors to inspect their responses honestly and to attempt to understand the origins and meanings of their reactions in their care of a patient, since this can lead to a better understanding of the patient's suffering. The role of supervision for clinicians is important in this regard. Fortunately, the ethical code prohibits certain actions on the part of the doctor. In the absence of these prohibitions, the doctor's countertransference feelings about patients could put the public in grave danger.

Psychiatrists particularly, and especially those who are involved in treating difficult and chronically suicidal patients, are not infrequently confronted with private thoughts that it would be good for all concerned if the patient did in fact successfully commit suicide. We also know that when we do have such feelings about a patient, it is a very reliable clinical indicator that the patient is indeed dangerously suicidal and needs our help more rather than less. This is the nature of the phenomenon of projective identification.

What psychiatrists confront with their individual patients, particularly the chronically suicidal and those with long-term disability and disorders like schizophrenia, is also faced by doctors in medical and surgical wards when treating patients with incurable disorders, and more so when there is an empathic gap between the doctor and patient based on education, wealth, class, ethnic background, or age. The situation is compounded by economic imperatives in the delivery of health care with restrictions on how long the patient can stay in the hospital, increased demand for a restricted number of hospital beds, and the lack of financial reward or personal psychological reward in looking after patients with poor outcome. Negative countertransference reactions from the doctor, whether recognized by him or her as such or not, can include hatred and murderous feelings (Gabbard 1996; Winnicott 1949), and these feelings may be inadvertently reinforced and encouraged by economic and managerial imperatives. Voluntary euthanasia, if legalized, would be more likely to be rewarded economically by third-party providers or government than palliative care. A number of authors have drawn attention to the influence of managed care in the United States on the doctor-patient relationship, particularly in a context in which physician-assisted suicide is debated (Caine and Conwell 1993), and the impact of health management practices on the issue of countertransference (Rao et al. 1997). An economic imperative for cost-effectiveness, coming as a directive from a managed care organization or health administrators, could easily be used to rationalize countertransference enactments in the form of physician-assisted suicide.

Preventing suicide and treating those who have attempted suicide is expensive and time-consuming. Legalizing assisted suicide allows society to offer suicide as an inexpensive treatment alternative. This is not as far-fetched as it sounds. The Dutch experience in this regard is of more than passing interest (Hendin 1994; Sheldon 1995). A psychiatrist in the now-famous Assen case assisted in the suicide of a female patient who had no physical illness but suffered from long-term depression and, if accounts of the history of the patient are correct, was driven to seek euthanasia by the death of one of her sons through cancer and the death of her other son by suicide some years earlier (Hendin 1994). Because this was outside the euthanasia guidelines that had been the practice in the Netherlands for some time with respect to patients with terminal illness, the doctor was charged by the authorities. However, the Dutch Court, while critical of some aspects of the doctor's conduct, held that what was done was consistent with Dutch euthanasia practice and that psychological suffering could not be distinguished from physical suffering for the purposes of euthanasia.

From a psychological point of view, the decision of the Dutch Court seems correct. The degree of psychological suffering experienced by some of our patients with schizophrenia, profound personality disorders, or, indeed, chronic depression is just as profound as that of patients with severe physical disorders including severe pain, although the nature and quality of the suffering are different. Moreover, the suffering from psychiatric disorders is not as easily ameliorated by the use of narcotics or other palliative care measures. It is also erroneous to delineate emotional and physical suffering as if the experience of an individual could be readily separated into these discrete domains (Cassell 1982; Kleinman 1995). If the extent of human misery is an issue, the arguments in favor of voluntary euthanasia and assisted suicide for patients with psychiatric disorders seem more powerful than the arguments in favor of those with terminal physical disorders, who we know can benefit from good palliative care in terms of amelioration of personal suffering.

So far in this chapter we have argued that the wish to kill on the part of the doctor—or to put it more mildly, the doctor's wish to go along with the wishes of the patient to die—is a reflection of the feelings generated in the doctor-patient relationship. The doctor's wishes, unconscious though they may be, may have their source in the patient's suffering and may thus be a reflection of this suffering; in other words, the doctor's feelings are a manifestation of projective identification (Sandler et al. 1992). We understand projective identification as a process whereby the patient, through projection of internalized good and bad objects into the doctor, compels the doctor to behave toward the patient or the patient's objects in a particular way. Countertransference in this model can be understood as a patient-induced response in the doctor that conforms to one of the patient's internal self or object representations (Gabbard 1995). However, such a view of what is going on in the doctor runs the risk of blaming the patient for the doctor's countertransference. An alternative view is that the doctor's feelings toward the patient, including destructive feelings, are what is brought to the clinical situation and indicative of pathological aspects of the doctor's psychological makeup—that is, countertransference as originally conceptualized by Freud (Sandler et al. 1992).

The developing view of countertransference as an intersubjective phenomenon involving the interaction of two persons in the clinical situation as articulated by Gabbard (1995) and others (Adler 1994) is particularly useful in understanding both the patient's wish to die and the doctor's reaction to and, indeed, role in this wish. Within this model, not only is countertransference seen as a spectrum encompassing projective identification on the one hand and countertransference enactment on the other, but the two are seen as interacting with each other. The model allows that the form in which the projective identification will manifest—that is, the manner in which a particular doctor will feel compelled to behave and act in a particular way toward a patient—is a function of what each brings to the interaction. In other words, not all therapists will have a particular reaction to a patient's projections, and the variance will be determined by unconscious factors operating in the therapist.

The intersubjectivity of countertransference phenomena is very nicely illustrated by the situation in which a patient requests assisted suicide. At one level, a patient's misery, suffering, and self-destructive impulses act to engender in the doctor feelings of disgust with suffering and death and a wish to terminate the patient's life. On the other hand, the patient's wish to die and the patient's self-concept as being worthless and a burden to others may in part be a reflection of what the doctor brings to the encounter (i.e., the doctor's omnipotent fantasies and disgust with death and decay or the doctor's inability to tolerate the patient's suffering). Thus, the doctor's wish to kill may be a major contributor to the patient's request. Similarly, the doctor's death anxiety may lead to an omnipotent need to triumph over death through physician-assisted suicide in order to preserve an illusion of mastery and control. This countertransference need of the doctor may subtly place pressure on the patient to choose euthanasia.

In this context it is valuable to examine the zeal with which some practitioners of euthanasia or doctors who advocate euthanasia pursue the cause of being allowed to terminate their patient's life. The Northern Territory legislation contained the requirement for a "cooling-off period" between the time the decision was made to request euthanasia and the carrying out of the act of termination of life by the doctor, which raises the question "Who is supposed to be cooling off?" We need to ask if there is not a certain aesthetic appeal, perhaps a relief of inner tension, or maybe even an emotional or intellectual satisfaction from playing on the edge of life and challenging traditional ethical stances that can drive certain doctors. Such a motivation, if present, is neither remarkable nor surprising if one considers the psychological factors that may operate in the choice of medicine as a career. There are certainly questions worth asking. What happens when a doctor's omnipotent fantasies about saving lives and defying death are thwarted by the inexorable process of incurable disease? Does such thwarting of fantasies result in the doctor's desiring the death of the patient and the elimination of the patient as a reminder of his or her impotence? We also need to ask whether the wish to cure and the wish to help represent a disguise for less comfortable and darker motivations. As Karl Menninger (1957) noted, the practice of medicine affords a unique opportunity to conceal conscious or unconscious sadism. As doctors, we place a high value on health and well-being. Does this translate into the disgust of decay and disease and deterioration?

Doctors who are faced with the decision of whether to accede to a patient's request for assisted suicide if it were legal, and psychiatrists or psychologists who are assessing the patient from the point of view of the patient's competency to make such a request, need to be particularly aware of their own response to the patient and the impact of the patient's suffering and what that means to them as doctors. Soul searching is important in any boundary crossing, let alone a major boundary violation (Gutheil and Gabbard 1993). Unfortunately, advocacy of euthanasia and assisted suicide as the patient's "right" in terms of ideology about autonomy tends to overshadow any examination of the subtlety of the doctor-patient relationship. This ideological blind spot may make advocates of euthanasia particularly unsuited to making decisions regarding the end of life.

It is of interest that when one examines traditional medical professional codes from whatever culture, these codes do not set out so much what doctors shall do, but rather what they shall not do—that is, they constitute a set of prohibitions. One of these prohibitions is that of doctors' taking life. It is as if when these codes were developed, there was perhaps an intuitive understanding on the part of those who developed them that one who could save life might also take it, and perhaps even that those who want to save life may wish to take it. A patient's wish to die is one thing, but the doctor's wish to kill is another.

Conclusion

The empirical evidence from studies of terminally ill patients indicates that the request for euthanasia and suicidal ideation and behavior occur in the context of complex clinical situations. In addition to paying attention to undiagnosed and untreated psychiatric disorder, the physician involved in the care of the dying patient needs to pay attention to the social and interpersonal context of the request for assisted suicide. Central to the context is the doctor-patient relationship, since the empirical evidence suggests that this has a profound effect on the patient's perception of his or her situation. A doctor's ability to understand the full context of the patient's end-of-life dilemma is severely compromised by the removal of the prohibition against killing, one of several prohibitions that form the therapeutic frame that allows the doctor-patient relationshp to function. It is not possible to assess "competence" to decide about euthanasia, because the question is outside the therapeutic frame. The expressed wish to die on the part of the patient may be a reflection of issues in the doctor-patient relationship that can be understood in terms of transference, projective identification, and countertransference enactment within an intersubjective model. Psychopathological factors in the doctor, including reactions to illness, death, and the failure of treatment, can influence the dying patient's end-of-life decision.

References

Adler G: Transference, countertransference, and abuse in psychotherapy. Harv Rev Psychiatry 2:151–159, 1994

Allebeck P, Bolund C: Suicide and suicide attempts in cancer patients. Psychol Med 21:979–984, 1991

Annas GJ: Physician-assisted suicide: Michigan's temporary solution. N Engl J Med 328:1573–1576, 1993

Baile WF, DiMaggio JR, Schapira D, et al: The request for assistance in dying: the need for psychiatric consultation. Cancer 72:2786–2791, 1993

Bindels PJE, Krol A, van Ameijden E, et al: Euthanasia and physician-assisted suicide in homosexual men with AIDS. Lancet 347: 499–504, 1996

Breitbart W: Suicide in cancer patients. Oncology 1:49–53, 1987

Breitbart W: Cancer pain and suicide. Advances in Pain Research and Therapy 16:399–412, 1990

Breitbart W: Suicide risk and pain in cancer and AIDS patients, in Current and Emerging Issues in Cancer Pain: Research and Practice. Edited by Chapman CR, Foley KM. New York, Raven, 1993, pp 49–65

Breitbart W, Rosenfeld BD, Passik SD: Interest in physician-assisted suicide among ambulatory HIV-infected patients. Am J Psychiatry 153:238–242, 1996

Brody H: Assisted death—a compassionate response to a medical failure. N Engl J Med 327:1384–1388, 1992

Brown JH, Henteleff P, Barakat S, et al: Is it normal for terminally ill patients to desire death? Am J Psychiatry 143:208–210, 1986

Caine E, Conwell Y: Self-determined death, the physician, and medical priorities: is there time to talk? JAMA 270:875–876, 1993

Cantor JC, Baker LC, Hughes RG: Preparedness for practice: young physicians' views of their professional education. JAMA 270:1035–1040, 1993

Cassell EJ: The nature of suffering and the goals of medicine. N Engl J Med 306:639–645, 1982

Cherny NI, Coyle NI, Foley KM: Suffering in the advanced cancer patient: a definition and taxonomy. J Palliat Care 10:57–70, 1994a

Cherny NI, Coyle NI, Foley KM: The treatment of suffering when patients request elective death. J Palliat Care 10:71–79, 1994b

Chochinov HM, Wilson KG: The euthanasia debate: attitudes, practices and psychiatric considerations. Can J Psychiatry 40:593–602, 1995

Chochinov HM, Wilson KG, Enns M, et al: Desire for death in the terminally ill. Am J Psychiatry 152:1185–1191, 1995

Chochinov HM, Wilson KG, Enns M, et al: Depression, hopelessness, and suicidal ideation in the terminally ill. Psychosomatics 39: 366–370, 1998

Clarke PJ: Exploration of countertransference toward the dying. Am J Orthopsychiatry 51:71–77, 1981

Commonwealth of Australia, Senate and Constitutional Legislation Committee: Consideration of legislation referred to the committee. Euthanasia Laws Bill 1996. March 1997

Conwell Y, Caine ED: Rational suicide and the right to die: reality and myth. N Engl J Med 325:1100–1102, 1991

DiMaggio JR: Educating psychiatry residents about death and dying: a national survey. Gen Hosp Psychiatry 15:166–170, 1993

Duckworth KS, Kahn MW, Gutheil TG: Roles, quandaries and remedies: teaching professional boundaries to medical students. Harv Rev Psychiatry 1:266–270, 1994

Fogel BS, Mor V: Depressed mood and care preferences in patients with AIDS. Gen Hosp Psychiatry 15:203–207, 1993

Gabbard GO: The role of compulsiveness in the normal physician. JAMA 254:2926–2929, 1985

Gabbard GO: Countertransference: the emerging common ground. Int J Psychoanal 76:475–485, 1995

Gabbard GO: Love and Hate in the Analytic Setting. Northvale, NJ, Jason Aronson, 1996

Gaita R: Reflections on the euthanasia debate. Eureka Street 5 (March):22–27, 1995

Ganzini L, Lee M: Psychiatry and assisted suicide in the United States. N Engl J Med 336:1824–1826, 1997

Ganzini L, Fenn DS, Lee MA, et al: Attitudes of Oregon psychiatrists toward physician-assisted suicide. Am J Psychiatry 153:1469–1475, 1996

Glick SM: Unlimited human autonomy—a cultural bias? N Engl J Med 336:954–957, 1997

Goodwin JS: Mercy killing: mercy for whom? (editorial) JAMA 265:326, 1991

Gutheil TG, Gabbard GO: The concept of boundaries in clinical practice: theoretical and risk management dimensions. Am J Psychiatry 150:188–196, 1993

Heitanen P, Lonnqvist J: Cancer and suicide. Ann Oncol 2:19–23, 1991

Hendin H: Seduced by death: doctors, patients, and the Dutch cure. Issues Law Med 10:123–168, 1994

Hendin H, Klerman MD: Physician-assisted suicide: the dangers of legalization. Am J Psychiatry 150:143–145, 1993

Hirsch DJ: Death from dialysis termination. Nephrol Dial Transplant 4:41–44, 1989

Holland J: Cancer and suicide: less common and more predictable than we thought? (editorial) Ann Oncol 2:8, 1991

Jaspers K: General Psychopathology. Translated by Hoenig J, Hamilton M. Manchester, UK, Manchester University Press, 1963

Kelly B, Varghese FT: Assisted suicide and euthanasia: what about the clinical issues? Aust N Z J Psychiatry 30:3–8, 1996

Kelly B, Varghese FT: The emotional hazards of medical practice, in Medical Consultation Skills. Edited by Sanders MR, Mitchell C, Byrne GJA. Melbourne, Addison-Wesley, 1997, pp 472–488

Kelly B, Raphael B, Judd F, et al: Suicidal ideation, attempted suicide and HIV infection. Psychosomatics 39:405–415, 1998

Kissane DW, Bloch S, Burns WI, et al: Perceptions of family functioning and cancer. Psychooncology 3:259–269, 1994a

Kissane DW, Bloch S, Burns WI, et al: Psychological morbidity in the families of patients with cancer. Psychooncology 3:47–56, 1994b

Kissane DW, Bloch S, Dowe DL, et al: The Melbourne Family Grief Study, I: perceptions of family functioning in bereavement. Am J Psychiatry 153:650–658, 1996

Kleinman A: Writing at the Margin: Discourse Between Anthropology and Medicine. Berkeley, University of California Press, 1995

Kuhse H, Singer P, Clark M, et al: End-of-life decisions in Australian medical practice. Med J Aust 166:191–196, 1997

Marzuk PM, Teirney H, Tardiff K, et al: Increased risk of suicide in persons with AIDS. JAMA 259:1333–1370, 1988

Menninger KA: Psychological factors in the choice of medicine as a profession, Part II. Bull Menninger Clin 21:99–106, 1957

Miles SH: Physicians and their patient's suicides. JAMA 271:1786–1788, 1994

Modestin J: Countertransference reactions contributing to completed suicide. Br J Med Psychol 60:379–385, 1987

Moulin D, Latimer EJ, MacDonald N, et al: Statement on euthanasia and physician-assisted suicide. J Palliat Care 10:80–81, 1994

Muskin PR: The request to die: role for a psychodynamic perspective on physician-assisted suicide. JAMA 279:323–328, 1998
O'Dowd MA, Biderman DJ, McKegney FP: Incidence of suicidality in AIDS and HIV-positive patients attending a psychiatry outpatient program. Psychosomatics 34:33–40, 1993
Owen C, Tennant C, Levi J, et al: Cancer patients' attitudes to final events in life: wish for death, attitudes to cessation of treatment, suicide and euthanasia. Psychooncology 3:1–9, 1994
Pellegrino ED: Compassion needs reason too. JAMA 270:874–875, 1993
Quill TE, Cassel CK, Meier DE: Care of the hopelessly ill: proposed clinical criteria for physician assisted suicide. N Engl J Med 327: 1380–1383, 1992
Rajs J, Fugelstad A: Suicide related to human immunodeficiency virus infection in Stockholm. Acta Psychiatr Scand 85:234–239, 1992
Ramirez AJ, Graham J, Richards MA, et al: Burnout and psychiatric disorder among cancer clinicians. Br J Cancer 71:1263–1269, 1995
Ramirez AJ, Graham J, Richards MA, et al: Mental health of hospital consultants: the effects of stress and satisfaction at work. Lancet 347:724–728, 1996
Rao NR, Meinzer AE, Berman SS: Countertransference: its continued importance in psychiatric education. Journal of Psychotherapy Practice and Research 6:1–11, 1997
Rothwell PM, McDowell Z, Wong CK, et al: Doctors and patients don't agree: cross sectional study of patients' and doctors' perceptions and assessments of disability in multiple sclerosis. BMJ 314: 1580–1583, 1997
Rundell JR, Kyle KM, Brown GR, et al: Risk factors for suicide attempts in a human immunodeficiency virus screening program. Psychosomatics 33:24–27, 1992
Ryan CJ: Velcro on the slippery slope: the role of psychiatry in active voluntary euthanasia. Aust N Z J Psychiatry 29:580–585, 1995
Ryan CJ, Kaye M: Euthanasia in Australia—the Northern Territory Rights of the Terminally Ill Act. N Engl J Med 334:326–328, 1996
Sandler J, Dare C, Holder A: The Patient and the Analyst: The Basis of the Psychoanalytic Process. Madison, CT, International Universities Press, 1992, pp 81–98
Schaerer R: Suffering of the doctor linked with the death of patients. Palliat Med 1:27–37, 1993
Seigel K: Rational suicide: considerations for the clinician. Psychiatr Q 54:77–84, 1982
Severson KT: Dying cancer patients: choices at the end of life. J Pain Symptom Manage 14:94–98, 1997
Sheldon T: Reprimand for Dutch doctor who assisted suicide. BMJ 310:894–895, 1995

Slevin ML, Stubbs L, Plant HJ, et al: Attitudes to chemotherapy: comparing views of patients with cancer with those of doctors, nurses, and general public. BMJ 300:1458–1460, 1990

Storm HH, Christensen N, Jensen OM: Suicides among Danish patients with cancer: 1971 to 1986. Cancer 69:1507–1512, 1992

Thomas L: Dying as failure. Annals of the American Academy of Political and Social Science 447:1–4, 1980

Uhlmann RF, Pearlman RA: Perceived quality of life and preferences for life-sustaining treatments in older adults. Arch Intern Med 151:495–497, 1991

van der Maas PJ, van Delden JJM, Pijeneborg L, et al: Euthanasia and other medical decisions concerning the end of life. Lancet 338: 669–674, 1991

Varghese F: The phenomenology of psychotherapy. Am J Psychother 42:389–403, 1988

Viswanathan R: Death anxiety, locus of control and purpose in life of physicians. Psychosomatics 37:339–345, 1996

Whippen DA, Canellos GP: Burnout syndrome in the practice of oncology: results of a random survey of 1000 oncologists. J Clin Oncol 9:1916–1920, 1991

Winnicott DW: Hate in the countertransference. Int J Psychoanal 30: 69–75, 1949

Zalcberg JR, Buchanan JD: Clinical issues in euthanasia. Med J Aust 166:150–152, 1997

Afterword

Glen O. Gabbard, M.D.

The five chapters in this book can provide no more than a sampling of how the concept of countertransference can be useful in psychiatric practice. As a group, they convey a message that must not be ignored—namely, that we cannot transcend who we are. Much of the emphasis in recent years on cross-cultural issues in psychiatry is closely related to this point. Although we evolve out of a specific genetic substrate, we are acted on by a set of environmental factors that are perceived and elaborated with idiosyncratic meanings unique to the individual's psychological makeup. As psychiatrists, we bring all of this subjectivity to each patient we treat and to each setting in which we work.

Another message of these chapters is that no clinician exists in isolation. Mutual influences occur between patient and psychiatrist throughout each interaction. A patient who makes the doctor feel sympathetic toward him may influence the doctor to provide a diagnosis other than antisocial personality disorder, even if the patient's history and symptoms clearly suggest psychopathy. A patient whose clinical condition warrants electroconvulsive therapy may not receive it because the doctor is unconsciously feeling guilty about his potential to enact his repressed and conflicted feelings of sadism toward the patient. A violent patient may be so terrorizing that the clinician cannot think clearly enough to prescribe a reasonable treatment plan. The variations are as infinite as human experience.

A common theme in the contributions in this book is the notion that we can never be entirely certain how our unconscious reactions to the patient are affecting clinical judgment. This fact of clinical practice suggests that we should be open to consultations with our colleagues whenever we are encountering difficulty with a patient. Many practitioners feel a sense of obligation to solve all clinical problems themselves. The phenomenon of countertransference reminds us that we all need to preserve a sense of humility and recognize that we need to rely on each other for help when we encounter complex clinical dilemmas. One of the reasons that psychotherapy is helpful is that a therapist can observe things about us that we ourselves do not see. The same principle applies to consultation. We all have our countertransference blind spots. A colleague who is removed from the therapeutic fray is often in a much better position to detect those areas of difficulty than we are.

Index